Facing the Complexities of Women's Sexual Desire

Facing the Complexities of Women's Sexual Desire

Vera Sonja Maass

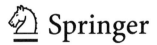 Springer

Vera Sonja Maass
Living Skills Institute, Inc.
Indianapolis, IN 46240-2366
USA
livskill@iquest.net

Library of Congress Control Number: 2006923103

ISBN-10: 0-387-33168-9   e-ISBN-10: 0-387-33169-7
ISBN-13: 978-0387-33168-3   e-ISBN-13: 978-0387-33169-0

Printed on acid-free paper.

9 8 7 6 5 4 3 2 1

springer.com

Preface

This book represents a broad-based approach to a narrow but complex issue. The issue causes distress for many and has been instrumental in family disruption and divorce. Women's sexual desire—whether it is too little or too much—has become an issue of growing concern and vague promises for solution. In the meantime, the women are looking for answers, consulting professionals in the field of human sexuality, physicians or therapists, media advice and self-help books.

The material discussed in this book is not part of any structured research. The women encountered in the pages of this book have not been selected on a random basis. Some have been clients, some are volunteers from the general population and another group is made up of undergraduate college students. The college students came from a varied ethnic and cultural background while the clients mainly were of white and African American background. The volunteers were predominantly from a white middle-class population. There is no claim that the women are representative of all women in the general population.

Some of the stories (Wilma & Nellie, chapter 2; Cindy & Jenny, chapter 3; Eileen, chapter 4; Karen, Jane & Nancy, chapter 5; Jeff & Libby, chapter 6; Mary, chapter 7; Robert, chapter 9) are based on materials discussed in "Taking Control of Your Life" or "Single Again" personal growth groups that were offered to the general public. Others (Louise & Jenny, chapter 3; Marian & Denise, chapter 6) have been part of class discussions in psychology and human sexuality courses. Their names have been changed and their circumstances disguised for reasons of confidentiality.

Acknowledgements

This book took on a different scope during a stimulating conversation with Janice Stern, Editor, Health and Behavior at Springer Science and Business Media, Inc. I am grateful to Janice for her interest in the project and her encouragement. Additional thanks go to Amanda Breccia, editorial assistant, who has made herself available for questions and has provided answers, and to Elizabeth Nesoff, editorial assistant, who has given new meaning to the term 'instant communication,' and to Allan Abrams, senior production editor, who was there to guide us through the complexities of the production phase of the book.

Tracy A. Dorsel, representative of the Procter & Gamble Company, who has shared the interest in women's sexual desire and who has been generous with pertinent information about the company's clinical trials and efforts to alleviate women's distress, deserves special thanks. Additionally, I want to express my appreciation to Cynthia Byer-Craney for her help with the women, who volunteered to share information from their lives.

List of Tables

Contents

Introduction

This book is written from the perspective of a sex therapist having listened to many of the complaints and concerns women have in relationship to sex. But only a segment of sexual difficulties are covered here, those difficulties that are examples of concerns in the desire phase of the sexual response cycle. These are issues of sexual aversion, hyperactive sexual desire, and hypoactive sexual desire.

The content of the book is organized into three main parts: Part I: Background and Explanations gives an overview of constraining influences on women's sexual experiences including historical-cultural constraints, pharmacological agents affecting women's sexuality, and physical-biological factors, such as the role of hormones, pregnancy and aspects of aging. A description of the three problem areas in the desire phase of the sexual response cycle follows. A summary of the various multidisciplinary exploratory efforts in search of explanations and answers to the complaints with focus on the promises and effectiveness of pharmaceutical as well as non-pharmaceutical approaches concludes Part I.

Part II has as its main focus the woman herself in the context of various aspects of life, beginning with women's search for personal and sexual identity, followed by sexual difficulties manifested in relationships, women's position in the dynamics of power and sexual desire, and intra-personal considerations and personality characteristics relevant to individual women's sexuality and the expression thereof.

Part III is a view towards resolution. Beginning with a brief historical account, early approaches in sex therapy that have laid the foundation for today's knowledge and work are discussed along with exploration of current therapies. The "Anxiety-Relief-Anxiety Cycle" illustrates the intimate connection between women's thoughts, feelings and consequent behaviors. The following chapter (10) focuses on a particular practical cognitive-behavioral treatment model. Various application modalities of the model, such as individual, conjoint, group, or single-sided relationship therapy sessions, are demonstrated. Finally, lessons from the past and thoughts for the future conclude the content of the book.

All through the book case histories and examples are used to highlight concepts as well as theoretical and practical concerns. The circumstances of the particular individuals have been disguised to protect their anonymity. Some of their stories have been combined to form composite characters. The women with their stories reflect a wide range of concerns common to many other women. The process of in-depth exploration of the contributing factors and search for increased pleasure and desire is a comprehensive one, involving various steps, which are described in detail.

Although the book is intended for use by professionals, such as sex therapists, sex educators, social worker-therapists, health psychologists, clinical psychologists, and advanced students in the mental health and human sexuality fields, the use of professional jargon has been avoided to make it accessible to readers not trained in psychology or counseling without watering down theoretical or professional concepts.

Therapists reading this book may feel they are recognizing some of their own clients in these pages and some female readers may derive comfort when they encounter other women struggling with concerns similar to their own.

PART I
Background and Explanations

1
Influences on Women's Sexual Experiences

More than 30 years after the so-called sexual revolution and the appearance of the "pill" on the contraceptive market, which afforded women a freedom of sexual activities previously enjoyed mainly by men, what are our current concerns about women's sexuality? Have the prophecies of doom and moral chaos as consequences of the feminist movement and the sexual revolution predicted by some, come to pass?

Historical Aspects

How lasting have the changes resulting from those movements been? Even a cursory examination of history reveals the enduring power of constraining influences on human sexuality in general and on women's sexuality in particular. These powerful influences continue to confront counter-movements that develop at different times and places in history. As the movements evolve, will they be strong enough to survive or will they crumble under the onslaught of the constraining doctrines of the past?

While the belief that women should be subservient to men remained strong throughout the Middle Ages, two contradictory images of women developed, each having a strong impact on women's place in society and on men's attitudes toward women. The image of the Virgin Mary was contrasted by the image of Eve, the evil temptress, who herself had succumbed to the temptations of the serpent in the Garden of Eden. The church's emphasis on Eve's sin culminated in the witch hunts that began in the late 15th century, and their traces can be detected in the so-called double standard that is still alive and well in many cultures.

There was a brief moment of enlightenment during the 18th century. Mary Wollstonecraft of England in her book *The Vindication of the Rights of Women* (originally published by Thomas and Andrews, Boston, in 1792) proclaimed that sexual satisfaction was as important to women as to men and that premarital and extramarital sexual activities were not sinful. These progressive views were soon buried by the attitudes and opinions of the Victorian era. Female sexuality was described in the quotations of the physician William Acton as something that did not bother the majority of women very much (Degler, 1980). As the roles for men and women were redefined, the worlds of men and women were separated, creating an emotional and physical distance between husbands and wives and male and female partners.

Alongside the prevailing notion of the asexual Victorian woman, prostitution flourished and afforded a livelihood for those who were not participating in the ladylike lifestyle of upper- and middle-class Victorian women. Celia Mosher, a physician born in 1863, conducted her own research of women's sexuality over a period of 30 years. In her surveys she found that the majority of women experienced sexual desire and orgasm (Ellison, 2000). Mosher's research started with a questionnaire developed by her for a lecture to The Mothers Club on the theme of "marital relations." Originally, the club consisted mostly of faculty wives at Stanford University, but she later also added information and data obtained from her patients (Bullough, 1994).

Of the 45 women who originally answered her questions, 35 stated that they felt a desire for sexual intercourse and 1 thought that sex was delightful. When asked about the "true purpose of intercourse," 9 women believed that intercourse was a necessity for men, but 13 of the women stated it was necessary for both males and females. Most of the women believed that the exchange of pleasure was a worthy purpose in itself. Several of the postmenopausal women reported still desiring and enjoying sexual intercourse. Many of the women had attended college and all of them were financially well off.

Cultural Constraints of the 19th Century and Beyond

Culture in the United States during the 19th century was full of sexual contradictions with women's sexuality being described in terms of opposing images of Madonna and whore. The psychological advances of the 20th century helped to expand the Victorian concepts about sexuality as researchers and writers expressed their views on human sexuality. Sigmund Freud reasoned that sexuality was as innate in women as it was in men. Havelock Ellis in his 1920 book *On Life and Sex* stressed the importance of "the love rights of women," and Theodore Van de Velde (1873–1937) in his popular marriage manuals emphasized the importance of sexual pleasure.

After World War II Alfred Kinsey's groundbreaking investigations into the sexual behaviors of American men and women were denounced by medical professionals, the clergy, and politicians; but his books *Sexual Behavior in the Human Male* (1948) and *Sexual Behavior in the Human Female* (1953) became best sellers. Almost 20 years later, with Masters and Johnson's works *Human Sexual Response* (1966) and *Human Sexual Inadequacy* (1970), women's capacity for orgasm was accentuated and sex therapy became a legitimate enterprise.

The media of the 1950s created a double-sided concept of sexuality for the American people. Television portrayed married couples in separate beds with at least one foot of distance between them, while practically at the same time the first issue of *Playboy* magazine, which focused on sex as recreation, arrived on the scene. Women looked for their own sexual identity within the confusing dichotomy of the "pajama-packaged" wife and the scantily clad sex kitten.

During the 1960s and 1970s sexual norms of previous decades were confronted through the feminist movement and the "sexual revolution" after oral contraceptives (OCs) provided women with security about unwanted pregnancies and afforded them the freedom to pursue sexual pleasure. Books emphasizing women's sexual awareness, such as *For Yourself: The Fulfillment of Female Sexuality,* by Lonnie Garfield Barbach (1975/2000), and varied experimental sexual behaviors, such as *The Joy of Sex,* by Alex Comfort (1972), appeared on the market. In her book *Liberating Masturbation,* Betty Dodson (1974) viewed masturbation as a healthy and positive aspect of sexuality. "Sex is like any other skill—it has to be learned and practiced" (p. 13). But the 1976 Vatican's "Declaration on Certain Questions Concerning Sexual Ethics" described masturbation as an "intrinsically and seriously disordered act," and in 1993 Pope John Paul II condemned masturbation as morally unacceptable.

The increasingly tolerant public atmosphere experienced a turnaround with the diagnosis of the first AIDS cases in the early 1980s. But even before that, psychological mechanisms evolved restricting procreative behavior to promote reproductive success and to maintain male-dominated society's power and control; sex was to be regulated, especially among women (Brownmiller, 1975). But because of its strong appeal sexuality cannot be completely suppressed. By linking sex to love, particularly romantic love, sex has been altered and elevated into a state of qualified acceptance. In American society, sex has thus been legitimized when considered an expression of heterosexual romantic love (Laumann, Gagnon, Michael, & Michaels, 1994).

Throughout the 20th century and beyond, gender-role socialization has persistently shaped men's and women's behavior and with that their notion of sexuality. The traditionally stereotyped version of the independent and aggressive male finds its complement in the equally stereotyped version of the dependent and submissive female. In men, sexual aggression is often excused by referring to their uncontrollable sexual desire as the cultural stereotype of the angry young man and the teenage boy with hormones raging out of control. This excuses males from taking responsibility for their sexual aggressiveness and instead places on women the responsibility for resisting and curbing male aggressiveness (May, 1998). If the woman does not do her job of curbing the male's sexual insistence, the word "slut" is readily available for her indictment. These lingering cultural stereotypes have long-lasting, indeed, lifelong effects on both male and female sexuality.

Cultural Factors Shaping Sexual Desire

To demonstrate how cultural factors function in shaping sexual desire, Simon (1994) analyzed the relationship between cultural factors and the "representation of desire." Within this context Simon asserted that objects can best be described through the "logic of metaphor." Our culture contains powerful signifiers related to human sexuality, Simon hypothesized, "... each with the capacity to link erotic significance to more general and, in some cases, older desires" (p. 11). These powerful signifiers can be classified by "family values" representations, which are linked to Old Testament and Christian beliefs about sexuality and gender roles, and the erotic representations linked to the sexually explicit and saturated media in contemporary American society (Michael, Gagnon, Laumann, & Kolata, 1994).

Between these two extremes, there is room for modern versions of the Victorian era's attitudes concerning female sexuality. Attitudes about human sexuality fluctuate as to severity or explicitness in different regions of the United States. Melanie, who considered herself a typical southern woman—gentle, educated, and well-mannered—serves as an example. She and her sisters accepted their mother's teachings about a woman's sexual behavior and duties within a marriage. Following her mother's example of a good wife, Melanie seemed happy in her marriage to Gregory. A few years into their marriage, as part of Gregory's promotion within his profession, he moved Melanie and their young son to a town in the northern Midwest. Adjustment to the new environment was not easy for anybody, especially for Melanie, who missed her circle of friends. Gregory's new position offered many opportunities for travel and professional growth. The initial excitement about the promotion gave way to feelings of depression. Despite his professional success he felt like a failure at home.

When he initiated sex, most often she would go along with it, but she was not responsive. It did not take long for Gregory to realize that Melanie did not enjoy his lovemaking. She never seemed to be ready to initiate sex. When he asked her about it, Melanie admitted that she was not very interested in sex.

Melanie worked on establishing healthcare agencies for her family in their new surroundings. Her new gynecologist referred her to a local clinic for sexual dysfunction. Although embarrassed at first, in her session with a female sex therapist Melanie explained that sex was not something a woman of her middle-class background in her home state was expected to enjoy. It was a wife's duty to be available for her husband, but men in general seemed to make connections to another type of women for this particular activity. While women are expected to enjoy pleasing their men, they are not supposed to enjoy sex themselves.

Although she was living in the 21st century, Melanie's opinion seemed to come straight out of the beliefs and attitudes of the Victorian era. Gregory, on the other hand, did not share Melanie's opinion. He desired an emotionally and physically intimate relationship with his wife. To him, his wife was the center of his being.

Sexuality and Mate Selection

Human sexuality is a complex concept that includes many different elements. Its definition and meaning may vary from one individual to the next, from one gender to the other, and at different times even within the same individual. In addition to anatomical and physiological aspects, self-knowledge or self-concept, beliefs, values, attitudes, thoughts, and emotions are elements relevant to human sexuality. Most sexual behaviors occur in the context of interpersonal relationships with varying degrees of intimacy and duration.

Historically and traditionally, gender roles have endowed men with primarily dominant characteristics, and these dominant characteristics are still preferred by most women when choosing a mate. A successfully dominant male is expected to provide greater protection from other members of the same species as well as easier access to resources and food. Similarly, men's social status is an important variable in women's partner choices. Characteristics that culturally translate into power seem to be inherently desirable to many women.

The desirability includes sexual desire—at least, for the early period of the relationship. With the passing of time personal and behavioral characteristics may function to reduce sexual desirability. As pointed out by Geary, Vigil, and Byrd-Craven (2004), culturally successful men share certain personality traits, such as being arrogant and self-serving. Such personality traits over time erode emotional and physical intimacy and lead to reduction of sexual desire within the partner who becomes the target of these behaviors. This aspect will be explored in greater detail in Chapter 6, which deals with the dynamics of power and sexuality.

On the other hand, for women, age can be a limiting factor in expressing and experiencing sexuality. The common cultural image of a sexually or erotically appealing woman is that of a young, slim female who looks more like a girl than a woman. Our culture created and, by encouraging men to pursue much younger women, continually perpetuates this cultural stereotype. Divorced, widowed, or never-married women past a certain age face the difficulty of finding sexual partners within their own age range. A recent survey revealing that 34% of women were dating younger men may indicate a change in the pattern of the double standard of aging (Mahoney, 2003).

The "Double Standard" Revisited

The sexual double standard has been a focus of research since the 1960s. Initially, it was defined as permitting sexual intercourse prior to marriage for men but not for women. Gradually, over time, the notion of the double standard took on a conditional aspect: that is, women were not stigmatized anymore for engaging in sexual activities as long as they took place within a committed love relationship, while men were allowed to have as many sexual partners as they wanted.

An analysis of research on sexual attitudes (Oliver & Hyde, 1993) demonstrated that the historical double standard of sexual morality—which is central to the suppression of female sexuality mentioned earlier—was more strongly accepted by females than males, although more recently the gender difference in attitudes toward the double standard is believed to have greatly lessened. However, in their 1999 study Millhausen and Herold found that women still believed that women judge other females who had engaged in sexual activities with many partners more harshly than do men. Pointing to contemporary sexual norms, Kimmel (2000) emphasized that the sexual double standard still exists.

Men were almost six times more likely to embrace a hedonistic or "playboy" philosophy than women.

In a review of 30 studies published since 1980, Crawford and Popp (2003) discovered evidence for the continued existence of sexual double standards. In the first large-scale study of sexual double standards Ira Reiss (1967) focused on individuals' attitudes about heterosexual permissiveness within premarital standards. His sample consisted of students from five high schools and colleges in addition to 1,550 adults. Attitudes toward premarital sex were classified into four general categories: premarital abstinence for both sexes; double standard with males given a greater right to have premarital sex; permissiveness with affection, where premarital intercourse was considered acceptable for both sexes within a committed relationship; and permissiveness without affection, including sexual permissiveness for both sexes, regardless of emotional involvement.

The findings showed that 42% of the students endorsed premarital abstinence from sexual involvement. Permissiveness with affection was acceptable to 19% of the students compared with 7% who endorsed permissiveness without affection. The "double standard" category had been subdivided into an "orthodox" view (premarital sex permitted only for males) and a "transitional" view (premarital intercourse permitted for females only if they were in love or engaged to be married). The orthodox double standard was endorsed by 11% and a transitional double standard was agreed to by 14%.

The opinions of the adult individuals in the sample were more conservative: 77% endorsed premarital abstinence, some sort of permissiveness was allowed by 11%, and some degree of double standard was accepted by 9%. In both the adult and student samples, men were more likely than women to endorse double standards and women were much more likely than men to support abstinence.

At the time, Reiss (1967) explained that egalitarianism had not been achieved yet, but the orthodox double standard seemed to reflect a minority attitude. After analyzing the studies from 1981 to 2001, Crawford and Popp (2003) concluded that some social and ethnic groups within contemporary American culture still endorse the absolute double standard that prohibits sexual involvement outside marriage for females. Furthermore, current double standards are more subtle but perhaps equally effective as instruments of social control. "Contemporary double standards allow some women greater sexual freedom than in the past. However, these standards still represent a covert means of controlling women's sexuality by judging its expression more harshly than men's sexual expression is judged" (p. 23).

In a study of 403 female general psychology students at the University of Kansas, Muehlenhard and McCoy (1991) explored the relationship between women's acceptance of the double standard (and their rating of their partners' acceptance) and the women's readiness to express their willingness for sexual desire. The students' ratings on the Sexual Double Standard Scale showed that the women thought that men believed in the double standard even more so than the men reported. Women who did not acknowledge their own desire for sex were more likely to believe that their partners adhered to the double standard than the women who were willing to openly admit their desire for sex. The researchers pointed out that the sexual double standard places women in a double bind. To preserve their "reputation," it is safest for them to be reluctant to acknowledge their own sexual desire, because if they do, they risk being negatively labeled.

These differential views of women and men's sexual activity can seriously affect the lives of women. When greater sexual experience on the part of a woman is regarded as negative and she is labeled with derogatory terms such as being "loose" or a "slut," many women may choose to appear as less experienced than they are to avoid harsh social judgment. This avoidance may be expressed in being unprepared for sexual intercourse—for instance, not having a condom handy for the man to wear. The consequences of this "innocence" can be extremely costly in terms of pregnancy or contracting a sexually transmitted disease.

In addition, women may internalize the double standards and evaluate themselves on the basis of them. This conformity to societal-based standards of morality may lead them to resist their own sexual desires. Cultural factors, such as the sexual double standard and general attitudes about sex, have significant impact on women's sexual interest.

Mass Media and its Impact on Female Sexuality

Quite different from the television programs of the 1950s, current American popular culture and mass media appear to promote a sexual ideology that is characterized by pleasure (DeLamater, 1989), victimization, and pain. The media has experienced increasing sexualization. In advertising, sexual images trivialize sex by proving that sex sells whatever is packaged in young, hard-body wrapping. When television news focused on the Clinton–Lewinsky scandal, new territory was charted with the use of the word *penis* and references to oral sex. Discussions about erectile dysfunction by Bob Dole were aired in promotional advertising of Viagra.

Popular soaps include sex acts on the average of six to ten per hour, depending on the show, involving sexual intrigue based on infidelity, revenge, and exploitation (Greenberg & Busselle, 1996). Some realistic information about sexuality and responsibility is brought into the television industry through cooperation with the Media Project, which also sponsors the annual SHINE Awards (Sexual Health In Entertainment) for programs that constructively portray sexual health issues (Folb, 2000). But, in general, the media rarely portrays sexually responsible models. TV programs repeat the myths and values, the facts and relationship patterns that define the social order, according to Cultivation Theory; and—based on Cognitive Social Learning Theory—the behaviors of the actors and actresses will be imitated by the people who watch the TV shows, especially those behaviors that find rewards rather than punishment in the plot (Brown, 2002).

Another issue is the manner in which female sexuality is represented in music videos. Apparently, in attempting to stimulate or satisfy the most stereotypical and immature male fantasies, big-breasted women are presented who seem to be in a constant state of sexual arousal and craving sex with irresistible but aggressive males. The extreme degree of depersonalization of these women is emphasized with the newest filming techniques. As the camera sweeps over disconnected body parts, the lyrics full of violent images as metaphors for sexual activity complete the scenario. The main function of these music videos with violence-saturated sexual images is to sell CDs and tapes. The videos are aimed at young people because they constitute the biggest buyer group. Exposure to the extreme stereotypical images in music videos could create or confirm gender antagonism in young people (Samuels, Croal, & Gates, 2000).

All these cultural and social influences have a way of perniciously invading the personal sphere of women's sexuality—their attitudes, beliefs, and values. Because the influence is so insidious, women often are not aware of the origins of their attitudes even as they fall victim to them. And because they are not aware of how these influences affect their personal lives, the women are not inclined to challenge their validity and replace them with more self-enhancing beliefs and attitudes.

Women's Views of Love and Sex: Resulting Attitudes

Men and women have different views of sex and love. Conventional wisdom has it that most women consistently seem to associate love with sex, whereas for men it is easier to have sexual intercourse for pleasure and physical release, without an emotional commitment. For men the main goal for engaging in sexual intercourse is to experience pleasure and physical release. Deep emotional commitments are not always a part of a man's sexual activities. Women, however, view sex as a purposeful activity that eventually leads to motherhood. Love and emotional commitment are necessary factors intertwined with sex. For men, after having fathered some offspring, procreation is not a main objective; pleasure appears to be a legitimate goal for sexual activities.

However, both men and women proclaim to value love and affection in sexual relationships. But men often avoid physically expressed affection because it may give rise to suspicions of being homosexual or—at the least—of being weak. For those women who consider being held for a while after lovemaking an important expression of affection, but have lovers who turn around and go to sleep after sex, there are moments of loneliness and disappointment in the aftermath of sex. It is not difficult to imagine that the disappointment is not conducive to increasing these women's interest in future sexual activities. In fact, this disappointment often gives rise to the notion that the woman's body has been used solely for the man's physical satisfaction.

Men and women also have different—and at times ill-defined—ideas about how long a couple should wait before engaging in sexual relations. Female students in a Human Sexuality class reported that their boyfriends usually pushed for sex before they wanted to engage in it. When asked about the length of dating time they would consider appropriate before entering into a sexual relationship, most of them stated "at least a month," but several added "it depends on the feelings I have for the guy."

Fear of Losing a Relationship

Many dating relationships—especially among the very young—begin with a false perception by both partners that their peers are having sex much more quickly than they are, partly due to common media implications. Social expectations of "instant sex" can present a challenge to those who want to move gradually into a sexual relationship. It is a pressure that may lead some individuals to a hasty start into a problematic sexual relationship. Often the fear that the other person will withdraw from the relationship if sex does not become part of it will prompt a young woman to agree to engage in sexual activities earlier than she originally believed would be appropriate for her.

Fear of loss can become a motivating force and for a while this fear can activate a certain degree of passion in a person; however, on a continuing basis, fear is not a healthy motivator. In the long run, performing activities out of fear will add negative aspects to the activities until they become as dreaded as the loss of what they were designed to prevent. It becomes a vicious cycle: engaging in sex out of fear of losing a valued relationship eventually frames the relationship in negative terms. The person who initially values the relationship experiences the activity that is required to prevent its loss as emotionally negative as the loss itself.

Pharmacological Agents Affecting Sexual Functioning

Psychiatric medications, such as some antidepressants, can affect individuals' sexual responses; there may be reduced sexual interest and arousal and delayed or absent orgasm. Some tranquilizers can interfere with orgasmic response. Similarly, medications prescribed for high blood pressure can interfere with sexual desire, arousal, and orgasm. Prescription gastrointestinal and antihistamine medications can have an effect on desire and arousal functions. Some nonprescription medications, such as may be used for motion sickness and gastrointestinal problems, also have an impact on sexual functioning.

Antidepressants

Elevated serum levels of testosterone may be associated with premenstrual dysphoria. Women, who use selective serotonin reuptake inhibitors (SSRIs) during the premenstrual period to alleviate irritability may feel better with lower testosterone or higher levels of serotonin; however, the lower testosterone level can decrease sexual desire.

Some observational studies attempted to identify whether initial treatment with antidepressants was linked to sexual dysfunction. One study reported an incidence rate of 56.9% in women with no prior sexual dysfunction when they were treated for depression (Montejo, Llorca, Izquierdo, & Rico-Villademoros, 2001). A retrospective review of clinic charts on depression from patients who were referred from primary-care physicians and psychiatrists revealed a 13.8% incidence (Keller Ashton, Hamer, & Rosen, 1997). It was noted that older women and those who were married tended to experience greater sexual dysfunction. No differences in sexual dysfunction based on the type of serotonin reuptake inhibitor were found.

Psychotropic drugs—as mentioned above—can have a significant effect on sex receptors during any part of a woman's life (Saks, 2000). Medications such as · Effexor, Serzone, Wellbutrin, and Remeron are thought to cause less sexual dysfunction than drugs like Paxil, Celexa, Luvox, Zoloft, and Prozac. SSRIs, such as fluoxetine (Prozac), sertraline (Zoloft), paroxetine (Paxil), Celexa, fluvoxamine (Luvox), venlafaxine (Effexor), and tricyclic antidepressants seem to stimulate postsynaptic receptors in the spinal cord which result in inhibited orgasm and— at times—anorgasmia (Rosen, Lane, & Menza, 1999; Saks, 2000). These are important considerations when treating dysphoria in women.

Oral Contraceptives and Libido

Considering the use of birth-control agents raises the question of a linkage to women's desire for or interest in sex. Since the "pill" became available on the market more than 40 years ago, researchers have generally focused on the safety and efficacy aspects of oral contraceptives (OCs). Few studies have explored the impact of OCs on sexual functioning. Although sterilization is the most prevalent method of contraception; among young women, oral contraceptives are the most frequently used reversible method. In a review of 30 research studies involving oral contraceptives and possible effects on libido Davis and Castaño (2004) found that in 1995 about 10 million U. S. women reported current OC use.

Although oral contraceptives are used to treat a variety of painful gynecologic conditions, their primary use is to avoid unwanted pregnancies. But as fears of pregnancy can have negative influences on women's sexual interest (Graham, Sanders, Milhausen, & McBride, 2004), some questions about indirectly negative effects of OCs on women's moods have surfaced. However, several studies examining mood effects linked with use of contraceptives have not revealed significant effects on mood attributable to OC use (Graham & Sherwin, 1993; Leeton, McMaster, & Worsley, 1978; Redmond et al., 1997).

Common combination oral contraceptive pills contain ethinyl estradiol and a synthetic, orally active progestin; their main mechanism of contraception is the prevention of ovulation, which is accomplished through inhibition of the release of gonadotropin from the pituitary. In addition, there are other changes that occur. The estrogen in OCs induces an increase in hepatic production of serum hormone binding globulin (SHBG). Thus, during OC use, the increase in SHBG results in a 50% decreased level of free testosterone. In addition, OCs decrease the androgen production by the ovaries and adrenal glands (Rabe, Kowald, Ortman, &

Rehberger-Schneider, 2000). The reduced androgen environment due to OC use makes an OC-mediated effect on libido biologically plausible.

Studies Concerning Oral Contraceptives

Women may be forced to decide whether to be in control of the number of children they want to bear or to protect the level of their libido. Trading protection from unwanted pregnancy for lower levels of sexual desire can become a dilemma, and additional research is needed. In their review of studies reported in the literature Davis and Castaño (2004) distinguished between several categories, such as retrospective, uncontrolled; prospective, uncontrolled; prospective and cross-sectional controlled; and randomized, placebo-controlled studies.

Retrospective, Uncontrolled Studies

In this group of studies, variable changes in libido attributed to OC use were reported, ranging from large increases to modest decreases in libido. Studies that were conducted in the 1960s—soon after OCs became widely available—show larger libidinal increases; perhaps because they were the first effective contraceptive method and the women's relief of feared pregnancy resulted in greater interest in sexual activities (Goldzieher, Moses, & Ellis, 1962).

Prospective, Uncontrolled Studies

Among this group of studies was one which included all women starting OCs who presented to a family planning clinic. Measurements of libido were recorded at baseline and again in 6 months (Cullberg, Gelli, & Jonsson, 1969). According to the authors, no significant change was observed. But 5% of the women participating reported that their libido had decreased and thirteen women discontinued OCs before the end of the study, one of them because of "sexual symptoms." It should be kept in mind, however, that at the time of this study much higher doses of OCs were used than are prescribed today.

Another, more recent, study, involving women at a family planning clinic and a university health center utilized a structured interview and a sexual experience scale at baseline and at 3, 6, and 12 months thereafter (Sanders, Graham, Bass, & Bancroft, 2001). Of the 107 women enrolled, 26 were lost to follow-up, 2 became pregnant, and 8% of those who discontinued or changed OCs gave "sexual side effects" as reasons for change.

Prospective and Cross-Sectional Controlled Studies

In these studies, the OC users' experience of libido is compared to that of another group of women who are not using OCs. Women starting with one of three different OCs were compared to a group of intrauterine device (IUD) users

(Herzberg, Draper, Johnson, & Nicol, 1971). Of the women in this study, 44% discontinued OCs, with 19% of them giving loss of libido as a reason. Comparing continuing OC and IUD users, Barnard-Jones (1973) found that more women in the OC group reported decreases in libido than in the IUD group.

Volunteer undergraduate students made up another group of participants in a cross-sectional design study attempting to determine the effect of OCs on libido by comparing established OC users to non-OC users (Bancroft, Sherwin, Alexander, Davidson, & Walker, 1991a, 1991b). Validated questionnaires were used in combination with sexual motivation measures based on a sexual experience scale. The results indicated that the OC users had higher sexual motivation and higher sexual desire ratings along with *lower* free testosterone levels than the women who did not use OCs. But, apparently, the OC users were different in attitudes and behavior from the nonusers, and since these differences between the groups were not considered in the results, generalization of these findings may be limited (Davis and Castaño 2004).

Randomized Controlled Trials

This type represents the most efficient study design because both known and unknown confounding variables are controlled for by the randomization. In the largest study in this category (Cullberg, 1972), women who had not used oral contraceptives were randomized to one of three OCs or a placebo group and were instructed to use other contraceptive methods during the study. The content of the medication packets was not known to the participants nor the investigators. Participants reported some increases and decreases in libido during the study, but there were no statistically significant differences found between the different OC groups or between the OC and placebo groups.

In some of the reviewed studies, sterilized women or women with sterilized partners were included as participants (Graham, Ramos, Bancroft, Maglaya, & Farley, 1995; Leeton et al., 1978), but again, generalization of the results may be difficult due to the variations in group composition. Overall, the randomized, placebo-controlled trials would be expected to provide stronger evidence than the other types of studies mentioned, but all of them include methodological limitations. The evidence currently available may indicate a small decrease in libido linked to OC use but it would be difficult to detect such a change within the context of OC use in the clinical research and within the women's subjective experiences.

The Role of Hormones

The significance of hormones in relation to sexuality is widely acknowledged. Testosterone, the dominant androgen in both males and females, is crucial to sexual interest and response in both men and women. It is important to realize that about 95% of the testosterone circulating in a man's blood system is bound (on a protein molecule) and therefore metabolically ineffective. In order to estimate the degree of impact testosterone has on an individual's sexual interest, one must look at the remaining amount of free testosterone, which is metabolically active and influences the libido. For males that is about 5%; and for females the free testosterone, which produces effects on bodily tissues, is only 1% to 3% of the total testosterone.

Reasons for Androgen Insufficiency

Androgen insufficiency in women has been found to be associated with hypopituitarism, adrenal insufficiency, ovarian failure, and oophorectomy. It is not necessarily a specific consequence of natural menopause but can occur as a secondary factor to the age-related decline in the adrenal and ovarian androgen production. It is important to keep in mind that birth control pills may also decrease the ovary's production of androgens; this is also the case for postmenopausal women who receive estrogen replacement therapy.

Screening for androgen deficiency is usually done through blood samples. There are some difficulties in assessing testosterone levels accurately because the methods used were originally developed for men, who generally have higher levels of circulating testosterone, as described earlier. The significantly lower levels of free testosterone in females impair the accuracy of the blood tests (Guay, 2002). Furthermore, there has been some disagreement about the possibility that testosterone production in women may not be diurnal, as it is in men. If variations exist, higher production would be expected to occur in the morning. Therefore, it would be recommended to draw blood for assessing testosterone levels in women during the morning hours, between 8 A.M. and noon. Massafra and coworkers (Massafra, De Felice, Agnusdei, Gioia, & Bagnoli, 1999) found that androgen production also seems to vary during a woman's menstrual cycle, with a peak toward mid-cycle. This would suggest that the period from day 8 to 18 of the menstrual cycle would be the most opportune time for measuring androgens.

Establishing Normal Levels

In attempting to establish normal levels of hormones such as androgens in women, the accuracy of research findings has suffered because of the selection criteria applied to women in control groups: i.e., the women in the control groups were not screened for sexual dysfunction. Hormone insufficiency is not the only causal factor in female sexual dysfunction and especially not in the occurrence of low sexual desire. It has been estimated that more than 40% of women between the ages of 18 and 59 years experience decreased sexual desire (Laumann, Paik, & Rosen, 1999). Detailed interviews and use of adequate questionnaires as part of the selection process are needed to explore the sexual interest levels and actual participation in sexual activities and to identify the possible existence of sexual dysfunction in the women of the control groups.

The Effects of Estrogen

Another important hormone in female sexual functioning is estrogen. During menopause less estrogen may result in decreased libido, irritability, sleep disturbance, and reduced lubrication. In pregnant women, estrogen levels are usually high, but postpartum they drop significantly as the placenta is removed. This drop in estrogen may cause vaginal dryness and a decrease in sexual desire. Additionally, breastfeeding can create high levels of prolactin postpartum, which can also reduce sexual desire (Minkin & Wright, 1996).

Sexual Interest During Pregnancy and Beyond

In several studies, pregnant women's levels of sexual interest were compared with those they experienced prior to the pregnancy. The proportion of women with reduced sexual desire ranged from 57% to 75% in the third trimester (Bogren, 1991; Sayle, Savitz, Thorp, Hertz-Picciotto, & Wilcox, 2001).

During the postpartum period, sexual interest is generally low after delivery (Barrett et al., 1999, 2000; Oboro & Tabowei, 2002), with reduced sexual interest at 3 months postpartum reported by 23–57% of the women, while at 6 months postpartum reduced sexual desire was found in 21–37% of women.

In an analysis of responses from 104 women obtained at 12 weeks postpartum and from 70 women at 6 months postpartum, it was shown that by 12 weeks postpartum, the majority of women had resumed sexual intercourse, although many of them reported experiencing difficulties with dyspareunia and lowered sexual desire (De Judicibus & McMabe, 2002). Several factors were associated with decreased sexual desire and frequency of intercourse. These included depression, fatigue, and lower relationship satisfaction. As would be expected, women who did not breastfeed reported fewer sexual difficulties than women who were nursing their babies. Even when the babies were already 6 months old, the women continued to experience significantly lowered sexual desire and reported decreased frequency of intercourse. The women seemed to experience a significant degree of depression.

Menopause and Sexual Functioning

The term "sexual functioning" is defined in this book as engaging in activities of a sexual nature, such as penis–vagina intercourse, oral–genital stimulation and pleasuring, anal penetration, and individual and mutual masturbation to the satisfaction of the individuals involved.

The effect of menopause on women's sexual functioning has been a concern for clinicians for quite some time as the underlying hormonal changes of the menopausal status are thought to have an adverse impact on sexuality. As the population of menopausal women is increasing due to the general increase in lifespan, sexuality after menopause has received greater attention. In the year 2000, approximately 42 million women in the United States were aged 50 years and older, and many of these women were postmenopausal. While the age of onset of menopause has not changed significantly, women's increased longevity is stretching the time they spend in menopause (Bachmann, 2004).

Clinical trials and surveys have attempted to provide information on the prevalence and types of sexual complaints associated with menopause. These research strategies focus mostly on hormonal effects on specific aspects of sexual functioning. As hormone production is linked to menopausal status, in most women sexual functioning becomes a function of aging. Another confounding variable relating to sexual functioning for both men and women is that of the length of the relationship (James, 1983) According to cross-sectional and longitudinal data, the frequency rate of sexual intercourse is reduced to about 50% over the first year of marriage compared to premarital frequency rates and is halved again during the next 20 years. Female sexual desire toward a partner can vary over time as can be seen in the Pillsworth, Haselton, and Buss (2004) study mentioned in Chapter 3. These confounding variables can introduce methodological problems when assessing the overall effects of menopause on sexuality (McCoy, 1998).

Analysis of cross-sectional data from the Melbourne Women's Midlife Health Project, involving a sample of 2,001 randomly selected Australian-born women aged between 45 and 55 years, showed that reduction in sexual interest was significantly linked with natural menopause rather than age or other factors (Dennerstein, Smith, Morse, & Burger, 1994). In their study, the investigators provided and compared results from surgical and natural menopausal women and those who had undergone oophorectomy. They found the highest rate of reduced desire in naturally menopausal women. The results of the longitudinal phase of the study revealed that women showed a significant decline in factors such as sexual responsivity, frequency of sexual activities, libido, and feelings for partner as the women passed through the menopausal transition. It should be kept in mind that androgen levels in this population of women were already low.

The authors attempted to determine whether sexual dysfunction caused distress in their female participants, but found an inverse relationship between scores on dysfunction scales and scores on the distress scale, revealing that not all women with low sexual-functioning scores seemed to be distressed. In a cross-sectional national probability sample survey of American women, Bancroft, Loftus, and Long (2003) found that 25% of the women reported significant distress about their own sexuality; even though older women more commonly experienced sexual problems, it was the younger women who were more likely distressed by them.

Sources of Distress Over Sexual Dysfunction

The missing link in this interpretation of women's distress over their sexual dysfunction may be the exploration of the sources of the distress. There are women who are not distressed about their own partner-oriented sexual inactivity. However, young women in a committed relationship may well become distressed over what is determined to be their sexual dysfunction because of the effect this has on their relationship with their partners who have maintained their interest in sex.

Because sexual complaints during menopause frequently involve vaginal dryness and dyspareunia, which are associated with low estrogen levels, estrogen therapy has been employed for the relief of menopausal somatic symptoms, such as hot flashes, night sweats, and vaginal dryness. However, it was found that low-dose estrogen combined with low-dose androgen proved more effective in reducing these symptoms than estrogen alone (Simon, 2004).

Confronting Androgen Insufficiency in Women

While estrogen therapy may reduce the somatic symptoms of menopause, it often does not provide adequate restoration of the woman's sexual desire. Several testosterone products originally developed for men have found application with naturally and surgically menopausal women with low sexual desire, although testosterone therapies have not been approved by the U.S. Food and Drug Administration for treatment of female hyposexual desire. The testosterone formulations used with women include products that can be administered orally as well as, implants, injections, and sublingual testosterone.

Transdermal patches, gels, and emulsions are either already available, in development, or under observation in clinical trials. More recently, though, a notice in the January issue of the AARP Bulletin (2005) entitled, "Cold Shower from FDA," reports that women hoping to be able to increase their libido with government-approved pharmaceutical assistance will be disappointed. *Intrinsa*, Procter & Gamble's testosterone patch, did not receive the hoped-for stamp of approval from the Food and Drug Administration. Apparently, further research involving "possibly longer clinical trials and stronger evidence of benefits" is required (p. 21).

Sexual functioning (as defined earlier) is affected by a whole range of variables of which hormonal factors are only one part. The woman's premorbid level of sexual functioning—her level of sexual activity prior to menopause—her personality, level of education, physical and psychological health status, and feelings toward her partner all affect her sexual interests. "Given the range of factors affecting sexual functioning and the variability of the impact of those factors on each individual woman, it is important to recognize that a hormonal prescription alone may not be sufficient to change sexual function" (Dennerstein, Alexander, & Kotz, 2003, p. 80).

Surgical Menopause and Sexual Functioning

Hysterectomy is the most frequently performed major gynecologic operation and there are reasons to suggest that female sexual functioning may be adversely affected by disrupting the anatomical connections in the pelvis as occurs with the surgical removal of the uterus (Maas, Weijenborg, & ter Kuile, 2003). The literal meaning of the word *hysterectomy* is "removal of the uterus." The surgical removal of both the uterus and the cervix is referred to as "total hysterectomy." *Oophorectomy* is the surgical removal of the ovaries at the time of hysterectomy.

Hysterectomies among most premenopausal women are performed for benign, i.e., non-life-threatening conditions, such as dysfunctional uterine bleeding and uterine fibroids, whereas among postmenopausal women most hysterectomies constitute a surgical treatment for a prolapse of the uterus. In the smaller number of cases where hysterectomies are performed because of endometrial cancer, the surgical procedure is more extensive.

In premenopausal women hysterectomy results in a hormone deficiency, which may lead to sexual dysfunction. The resulting decrease in estrogen may bring about lack of vaginal lubrication and with that painful intercourse; but it is the androgen deficiency that is indicated as the cause of reduced sexual desire and arousability. Because the main hormone production occurs in the ovaries, oophorectomies would not be expected to interfere significantly with continued hormone production. However, some of the evidence in the relevant literature seems to indicate that hysterectomy with ovarian conservation is associated with premature ovarian failure (Siddle, Sarrel, & Whitehead, 1987).

Considering the notion that androgens play a significant role in the level of sexual desire, androgen substitution appears promising (Ginsburg, Rosen, Leiblum, Caramelli, & Mazer, 2000; Shifren et al., 2000). A randomized controlled trial with physiological testosterone replacement in women over 48 years of age has shown significant improvement in the level of pleasure and orgasm capacity but not in the degree of desire (Basson, 2003).

Sexuality Following Hysterectomy

Sexuality after hysterectomy has been the topic of several studies. Farrell and Kieser (2000) undertook a systematic review of the literature and found that in many of the studies variables varied and were poorly defined. In particular, the areas of sexual interest and sexual fulfillment were left undefined. Responses to questions regarding the frequency of sexual intercourse were assumed to reflect the degree of sexual desire experienced by the women. Any sex therapist knows that the frequency of sexual activities is not a reliable measure of the felt excitement and desire. In addition, many of the authors did not inquire about the women's pre-hysterectomy sexual attitudes and experiences. Nor did the researchers consider the importance of such confounding variables as relationship with partner or general psychological well-being.

In a 2-year study involving 1,101 women in the state of Maryland, a general improvement rate of 60% in sexual activity was reported after hysterectomy. However, some women developed sexual problems after the surgery: 10% of women who did not have a problem prior to hysterectomy were not sexually active after the surgery, and among those who developed difficulties post-hysterectomy

5.2% developed low libido. Women who were sexually inactive pre-and/or post-hysterectomy were not included in the data analysis, and the authors cautioned that the reported percentages of sexual dysfunction could be an underestimate (Rhodes, Kjerulff, Langenberg, & Guzinski, 1999).

In a comparison of the effects of total versus subtotal abdominal hysterectomy in 279 women the authors of the study concluded that neither type of surgery resulted in adverse effects on sexuality (Thakar, Ayers, Clarkson, Stanton, & Manyonda, 2002). However, as pointed out by others (Maas, Kenter, & Trimbos, 2003), the analysis of this study was restricted to women who were sexually active before and after the surgery, which compromised the randomization because 30% in the total hysterectomy group were excluded due to cessation of sexual activity as compared to only 19% in the subtotal hysterectomy group.

Information about the reasons for the lack of sexual activity was not given. This again may indicate a general underestimate of sexual dysfunction after hysterectomy. Furthermore, the assessment instruments used were restricted to the existence of sexual and physiological function; emotional aspects, such as anxiety or depression, were not addressed. Thus, the best predictors of sexual satisfaction or distress, according to Bancroft and coworkers (2003)—general emotional well-being and the emotional relationship with the partner—were neglected in the analysis. Purely physical aspects of sexual response in women, such as measures of arousal, vaginal lubrication, and orgasm, appear to be inadequate predictors of women's sexual enjoyment.

Other Variables Associated With Sexual Functioning

The occurrence of sexual problems is associated with several other variables, such as age, relationship issues, physical and mental health problems, and socioeconomic conditions. Women with significant psychiatric problems prior to hysterectomy would be expected to have similar problems after the surgery. Similarly, women's sexual attitudes and thoughts before hysterectomy can be significant predictors of the level of sexual interest after the surgery. On the other hand, when levels of post-surgery sexual interest are compared to rates prior to surgery, an increase in sexual interest after surgery can be observed in cases where the woman was symptomatic and in need of corrective surgery.

The fact that the potential health problem is no longer a concern was suggested as another possible explanation for increased sexual interest post-surgically in women who were predominantly younger (Rhodes et al., 1999). It would not be surprising to observe an increase in sexual interest after women experience reduced anxiety about the needed surgery, particularly in cases where the women had a healthy sexual appetite prior to the existence of the condition that required the surgery.

Women are often subjectively not aware of the physiological measures of their arousal, and therefore these aspects do not impact significantly women's felt enjoyment in sexual activities. Although hormones play a crucial role in enjoying a healthy sex drive, an even more critical role in women's sexuality is implemented through the quality of the relationship the woman is involved in (Rhodes et al., 1999).

According to Elizabeth Lee Vliet (2005), author of *The Savvy Woman's Guide to Testosterone,* "Female sexual desire clearly has biological components stimulated by optimal estradiol and testosterone. For women to become fully sexually aroused, it is equally or even more important to have satisfying emotional-intimacy connections" (p. 219).

2
Desire-Phase Problems and the Search for Explanations

Early conceptualizations of sexual desire as clinical considerations to explain peoples' varying motivation to engage in sex are found in the work of Kaplan (1977) and Lief (1977). Since then, different theories about sexual desire and its varying experiences and expressions have evolved. It is important to remember that in order to be categorized as a disorder, any of the components of a sexual dysfunction needs to cause personal distress to the individual woman. This requirement is part of a revised definition of female sexual dysfunction as developed by an international group of professionals from ten disciplines related to female sexual health in congruence with the criteria outlined in the *Diagnostic and Statistical Manual of Mental Disorders* (DSM-IV-TR) (Basson et al., 2000). For instance, some women have low sexual desire, but their life circumstances are such that it does not cause them personal distress; and in these instances one would not regard the low libido as a disorder (Pertot, 2005).

Difficulties in the desire phase of the sexual response cycle are normally thought to include sexual aversion and hypoactive sexual desire. However, because hyperactive sexual desire—although perhaps less common than hypoactive sexual desire—also expresses itself in this phase, it will be discussed in this book. Sexual aversion disorder, a fear of sex and a compelling desire to avoid sexual contact, is a relatively rare problem and it is often the result of sexual abuse or trauma.

Sexual Aversion Disorder

This difficulty is also known as *sexual phobia* and *sexual panic disorder*. Individuals who experience this problem express anxiety, fear, or disgust when confronted with an opportunity for sexual interaction with a partner. Most often, such fears result from sexual trauma, such as rape or incest; some cases of sexual aversion may stem from a fear of intimacy or hostility toward the other sex, or, in some cases, from self-directed hostility.

Self-directed hostility can take many forms, from open self-hatred, combined with physical attacks on one's body, such as cutting, hair-pulling, etc.—although symptoms like those are often dealt with professionally under different diagnostic categories—to disliking one's body or body parts and hiding them from oneself or others for fear of ridicule, criticism, or even abandonment. This fear and anxiety about exposure can lead to the experience of physical symptoms in addition to psychological damage, as can be seen in the case of Wilma below.

Wilma: Fear of Abandonment

Wilma, a married woman with two children, had considered breast-reduction surgery before approaching sex therapy. Wilma has been in awe of her husband's intellect since their dating days. She met Rob, a chemical engineer, when she was 22 years old. As a teenager, Wilma had physically developed early; in high school her breasts were quite noticeable, while most of the other girls were still flat-chested. The self-consciousness she developed then stayed with her and was eventually reinforced when at the beginning of their relationship Rob mentioned his preference for women with a boyish figure and small, firm breasts. Wilma knew she did not fit that description. All the more grateful was she for his love, and over the years of their marriage she tried hard to please her husband in any way she could think of. Her pleasing behavior, which was based on her fear of abandonment, was the foundation of their marriage.

Wilma did not realize at the time that in the presence of her fear, the intimacy she desired could not develop. She was painfully aware of the fact that after giving birth to and nursing two children her breasts did not shrink in size. Instead of a participant in sexual activities she became a "spectator" or observer. Keeping her husband's original ideal picture of a woman alive in her mind, she was reminded on a daily basis of her own shortcomings. Displaying her naked body was extremely painful. She began to dread sex and tried to put it off as long as she could.

Rob complained about her reluctance to have sex. He thought he deserved more enthusiasm when he initiated sex. His criticism of Wilma's behavior increased and soon included other areas of their life, such as her cooking and how she disciplined their children. Not surprisingly, with every criticism her anxiety rose to new heights until she felt physically ill and nauseated at the thought of sex. Her family physician thought she had a sexual aversion disorder. Wilma never questioned why Rob had married her in spite of his preference for a female body quite different from her own. Was it perhaps in an attempt to establish control in their relationship from the beginning? In her gratitude for Rob's love she silently learned to dislike her body and become estranged from it. Was her body finally rebelling against her own dislike of it?

A therapeutic focus for Wilma would be to be on friendlier terms with her body and to recognize the importance of her body's function in giving and receiving pleasure through sexual activities. Relaxation exercises to calm herself down and reduce the high level of anxiety would be a valuable tool in coping with her situation. She would also need to separate her attitudes about herself from those of her husband, a task that could prove overwhelming to her.

Treatment for this condition involves providing insight and understanding of the origins of the sexual aversion. Opportunities for exploring and modifying negative attitudes associated with sexual issues combined with effective and open communication with the partner will be followed with sensate focus exercises to gently rebuild trust and self-confidence. In cases of a history of trauma, therapy dealing with trauma symptoms may need to be considered before focusing on the sexual aversion.

Nellie: Fear of Confinement

Nellie, a shy young woman, suffered from claustrophobia, which came to her employer's attention when Nellie refused to enter a small room where office machines, such as copiers and fax machines, were kept. The room had a door that could be locked from the outside. One of the older male employees attempted to calm Nellie down by placing his arm around her shoulders. Nellie screamed and forcefully pushed him away. Her employer valued Nellie's work and did not fire her, but referred her to psychotherapy instead. Nellie had not told anyone about her fear of locked spaces or where it originated.

In the therapist's office, Nellie disclosed what had happened to her during her brief marriage to an abusive man. In addition to the claustrophobia, Nellie also suffered from sexual aversion disorder. Mark, her former husband, had been very possessive of her. He did not want Nellie to go out by herself or talk to anyone. At first, she thought she did not have any warning signs about his abusiveness before they got married. However, as she talked, Nellie remembered an incident whereupon leaving a restaurant she noticed a female colleague with her husband at one of the tables. Nellie stopped for a brief greeting and wanted to introduce Mark, but he firmly gripped her arm and pulled her away, mumbling that they had to leave. Nellie had forgotten about the incident.

Soon after their wedding it became clear that Mark meant it when he told her not to talk to people in his absence. One day he came home from work and found Nellie talking on the telephone. Mark yanked the receiver out of her hand, slammed it down, and slapped Nellie's face. Nellie tried to defend herself but Mark did not listen.

Only a few days later, Nellie was in their clothes closet, looking for a particular garment. Suddenly, the door closed and she heard the noise of the key turning. Thinking that Mark had not been aware of her presence in the closet she called for him to let her out. He did not answer, although she was sure that he must have heard her. In the dark Nellie started banging against the heavy door. Then she heard steps toward the front door followed by the sounds of opening, closing, and locking the front door.

Nellie started yelling and crying hysterically but nobody heard her in the old building. Exhausted, she sank to the floor—shaking and whimpering for a while until she passed out. Several hours later Mark returned. He opened the closet door and jerked Nellie out of the closet. She could smell alcohol on his breath. As she tried to balance herself on her feet, Mark grabbed her, dragged her to the bed, and brutally raped her. Nellie waited for him to fall asleep, quietly got dressed, and left the apartment never to return.

Being afraid and ashamed, Nellie never told anyone about her brief marriage. The combination of the small appliance room in the office and the male employee's physical attempts to calm her down brought back her traumatic experience in full force. Nellie had not allowed herself to think about sexual issues after Mark had raped her. She was aware of her fear of small closed spaces and did her best to avoid them but she had managed to block out the rape. Now she had two issues to work on.

Hyperactive Sexual Desire Disorder

The acceptance of women's lower sexual desire as a biological fact, combined with the prevalence of female low-libido complaints in clinics involved in human sexual functioning and consequent discussion of this pervasive problem in the relevant literature, have led to relative neglect of those women who experience a high level of sexuality. We tend to focus on situations that present problems, so we can work on resolving them. While attending to the goal of solving difficulties that appear most pervasive in the public eye, we tend to overlook other, considered to be minor, difficulties. In the public opinion, highly sexual women may thus appear to experience minor difficulties.

According to Helen Singer Kaplan (1979), excessive sexual desire as a primary symptom constitutes a clinical curiosity because it is so rare. Kaplan cautioned that one must differentiate primary hyperactive sexual desire from high levels of sexual activity that are part of manic and hypomanic states. These individuals may respond to lithium therapy with a more manageable level of sexual desire in addition to a general calming.

Furthermore, compulsive and obsessive sexual states also need to be distinguished from true excessive sexual desire. These are individuals who are preoccupied with their sexuality and may masturbate to orgasm several times a day. These individuals seem to be anxious and tense and attempt to relieve their discomfort with sexual activity. Sexual activity for the relief of tension is a compulsion rather than truly overactive sexual desire.

There are women who desire more frequent sexual activities than their partners do. Some women may experience biologically determined higher levels of sexual desire; some may be in a relationship with men who for reasons of their own have a lower level of sexual desire. During the late 1970s, Lydia, an attractive widow in her 60s complained of "nervousness" when she made an appointment at a mental health center. Her nervousness turned out to be a high-level anxiety symptomatic of an obsessive-compulsive disorder. In her work, Lydia was overly conscientious; she worried for hours if she thought she had made an error. In her personal life she was equally compulsive, not being able to rest until all the dishes had been washed, the floors scrubbed, and the furniture dusted.

When asked why she did not retire from her job since it was so stressful due to her worries, she answered that she was afraid that if she did not have a job to go to, she would not get out of bed—not even to go to the bathroom. The picture she saw in her mind was of herself lying in a soiled bed permanently until her death. That picture was scary enough to send her straight to work.

Lydia had a romantic relationship with a male friend. One day—although highly embarrassed—she was able to confide in her therapist that she was suffering from a "sexual tension." Her friend could not keep up with her sexually and it turned out that she masturbated excessively. Lydia confessed that she had suffered from this sexual tension as long as she could remember, and she feared that she was an evil person who would go straight to hell after her death. She had never told anybody about it. When her therapist explained that her sexual tension seemed to be a characteristic of her obsessive-compulsive disorder, Lydia appeared relieved. With medication targeting the anxiety component and psychotherapy, Lydia's condition improved slowly.

However, one of the psychiatrists considered Lydia's masturbation compulsion to be characteristic of a hypomanic state and prescribed a trial with lithium. The change in medical treatment did not work for Lydia.

Hypoactive Sexual Desire Disorder

By far the most frequent problem occurring in the desire phase is that of hypoactive sexual desire disorder (HSDD), a sexual difficulty experienced by both men and women, but far more frequently occurring in women. Among those who seek sex therapy this is the most frequent complaint. People with this condition neither masturbate nor do they engage in sexual fantasy or thoughts. They avoid sexual activity as long as they possibly can.

Hypoactive sexual desire as a generalized, lifelong condition is rare. People more commonly develop HSDD at a particular point in their lives. Although it may originate from abusive personal experiences, more frequently it is a reflection of unresolved relationship problems. Women with low sexual desire usually report more dissatisfaction with their relationships than do women with other sexual problems, such as dyspareunia or anorgasmia.

Reasons for the relationship dissatisfaction can range from the woman's partner not behaving affectionately except when intercourse is expected to occur, to the couple not maintaining an atmosphere of romance and love in their relationship outside the bedroom, to ineffective communication which may invite misinterpretations, to a lack of attraction. It seems that women with HSDD often regard intercourse as an obligation they engage in reluctantly to fulfill their marital duties.

The Many Facets of Hypoactive Sexual Desire

Assessing the existence of hypoactive sexual desire is complicated by the fact that no clear criteria for determining "abnormal" levels of sexual interest have been established. Individuals vary greatly in the degree to which they want to involve themselves in sexual activities; and even within the same individual, levels of sexual desire change over time. Predictably, sexual desire decreases over time, especially in the absence of novel stimulation. Other terms that have been used to refer to this condition of low sexual interests are *inhibited sexual desire, low sexual desire, impaired sexual interest,* and *low libido,* among others.

Although we tend to expect a decrease in sexual desire in people who have been married for 20 or more years, desire problems are also experienced by newlywed couples as well as unmarried couples. It is not just boredom or advanced age that are the main reasons for reduced sexual desire; these difficulties can occur among couples of all age groups, and in fact, sexual problems are the main cause leading to divorce during the first 3 years of marriage. It is often difficult for people to admit that they are not all that interested in sex because in our sex-satiated culture, everybody is expected to love sex (McCarthy & MacCarthy, 2003).

In perhaps the earliest publication reporting on women with no interest in sex, Hite (1976) found that 1% of the women contacted indicated having no interest in sex. More than a decade and a half later Rosen and colleagues (Rosen, Taylor, Leiblum, & Bachmann, 1993) reported that in their study of middle-aged women attending a gynecologic clinic 15.1% had never been interested in sexual intercourse. Outcomes from the 1992 National Health and Social Life Survey estimated the number of women with low desire to be in the tens of millions, whereas reports from the 2000 Female Sexual Function Forum meeting showed that premenopausal women and postmenopausal women complained in almost equal numbers about decreased sexual desire (Vliet, 2005). Another nationwide sample, involving a total of 2,604 women, aged 18 and over, found that while 41% of the women felt that having a satisfying sex life was very important, 38% reported that their sex life was negatively affected by their lack of interest in sex (Berman, Berman, & Schweiger, 2005).

As these studies reveal, the number of women experiencing this difficulty is significant. In recognition of this fact, the major part of this book will be devoted to discussions concerning HSDD, with particular focus on emotional and psychological factors involved in the etiology and maintenance of the problem. Among therapists, sexual-desire problems are considered to be the most complicated sexual difficulties to treat (LoPiccolo, 2000). Therefore, it seems somewhat surprising to find books that, while asserting the importance of sex for women and promising to provide guidance for women in caring for their sexual selves (Foley, Kope, & Sugrue, 2002), have devoted only about 6% of their volume to the discussion of the topic of sexual desire.

In addition to reasons for the problem residing within one individual, as mentioned above, there are likely relationship issues that have come about because of strained interactions between the partners. For this reason it is worth mentioning that research has explored some medications with possible beneficial results for the treatment of low sexual desire.

The Search for Explanations and Answers

With the advent of effective treatments for men's sexual problems, the focus of sexual medicine and the pharmaceutical industry has shifted to researching potential ways to treat female sexual dysfunction. The statistics indicating the need for this attention are impressive: Based on an average life expectancy of 82 years, over the next two decades about 40 million women will enter menopause and spend about one-third of their lifetime in that condition. In addition, about half of the almost 600,000 hysterectomies performed each year in the United States will result in premature, i.e., surgical, menopause for women at a younger age than with naturally menopausal women (Kingsberg, 2005).

The most prevalent female sexual dysfunction is that of decreased sexual desire, or hypoactive sexual desire disorder (HSDD). It is generally agreed that contributing factors to this difficulty include physical, hormonal, emotional, and/or psychological aspects of an individual's life (Farrington, 2005).

Multidisciplinary Efforts

Exploratory efforts regarding explanations for the causes and resolution of HSSD are underway in many areas of research. Members of the medical–pharmaceutical field, ethologists (who focus on developmental aspects that emphasize genetically determined survival behaviors presumed to have evolved through natural selection), as well as socio-cultural and psychological theorists all are involved in the search for answers. Some explorations may involve researchers from several neighboring disciplines, whereas other efforts may remain within one particular domain.

As Stephen Levine (1997), a clinical professor of psychiatry, stated, "A narrow area like sexual desire should be broken down into its biology, psychology, cultural frameworks, pathology, research findings, theoretical formulations, clinical processes, and so on, and few of us middle-aged folks have enough workable memory left for such breadth and depth. Thank goodness for libraries!" (p. 13)

The Female Sexual Response Process

In exploring the nature of women's reduced sexual desire, many researchers and clinicians start as a basis of investigation with a general understanding of the female sexual response process (Farrington, 2005; Kingsberg, 2005; Lobo et al., 2005), beginning with the work of pioneer sexologists William Masters and Virginia Johnson and their linear four-stage model, which consisted of excitement, plateau, orgasm, and resolution. The model was the same for males and females, except that males experienced a refractory period following the four stages.

Later, in the 1970s, Helen Singer Kaplan (1979) proposed a three-stage model with desire as the first stage, followed by excitement and orgasm. The linear models seem to imply that people move progressively and sequentially through the phases; however, that is not the case for many women. Women may reach excitement and even orgasm without experiencing desire; and, on the other hand, they may experience desire and arousal without reaching orgasm (Whipple, 2002). Furthermore, linear models are not considering non-biological factors, such as pleasure and relationship aspects (Whipple & Brash McGreer, 1997).

Adding a circular model to therapist David Reeds' model, which consisted of four stages—seduction (including desire), sensations (with excitement and plateau), surrender (orgasm), and reflection (resolution)—Whipple and Brash McGreer (1997) implied that during the reflection stage, if the sexual experience was satisfying, it would lead to another sexual experience. If, however, the experience was not pleasant, the woman might not want to engage in another sexual experience. According to this model, it would then be important for the woman to have a pleasant or satisfying evaluation of the sexual experience while she is in the reflection phase. This aspect may deserve attention in a treatment approach.

Another circular model, the Basson (2002) algorithm, acknowledges the impact of numerous psychosocial and emotional issues, clarifying that for women the goal of sexual activity is not necessarily orgasm but personal satisfaction. Some practitioners prefer to use the Basson algorithm because it facilitates the understanding of the circular nature of women's sexual response. It relieves the women's fear that there is something wrong with them when their sexual responses do not occur in a linear manner as their male partners' are thought to do (Farrington, 2005).

Medical–Pharmaceutical Approaches

Medical researchers and practitioners are dedicated to finding answers to the following questions: (1) What is the nature of the of the problem? (2) What causes the problem? (3) How can the problem be corrected or, at least, be made manageable (with the help of medication, surgery, etc.)? Another question dealing with possible prevention of the problem might follow after obtaining the answers to the first three questions. Of course, this brief outline presents an oversimplification of the overall process but it will suffice for a general understanding.

A placebo-controlled study found that 60% of women and men treated with the antidepressant buproprion (Wellbutrin) showed improvement in sexual desire and response deficits compared to 10% in the placebo group (Crenshaw, Goldberg, & Stern 1987). Also, the over-the-counter steroid hormone DHEA, which is naturally produced by the adrenal glands, may have beneficial effects. At around age 30, the adrenal glands produce less DHEA, which might indicate that the supplement could have a positive effect. This was explored in another placebo-controlled study, using 50 mg of DHEA daily for 4 months, and results of increased sexual thoughts and sexual satisfaction were reported (*Contemporary Sexuality,* 1999).

The pro-androgen building blocks DHEA and DHEA-sulfate (DHEA-S) are produced mainly in the ovaries and adrenal glands, and also in the brain and in tissues like the skin, muscle, and fat tissue. Before they can activate androgen receptors, androstenedione, DHEA, and DHEA-S have to be converted to testosterone (Vliet, 2005).

Because most of the research on hypoactive sexual desire has focused on the condition in menopausal and postmenopausal women, attention was given to the role of hormones, as they usually decrease during this part of a woman's life. An emphasis on pharmaceutical studies emerged, as reduced availability of hormones, and especially androgens, was linked to reduced sexual desire.

Pharmaceutical Investigations: Viagra

The enormous success of the drug sildenafil, or Viagra, for erectile problems in men prompted Pfizer to consider Viagra's applicability for women's sexual difficulties. However, Viagra's function of increasing blood flow to the genital areas did not have the expected effect in women. Increased blood flow has a positive effect on sexual arousal but does not address women's sexual desire in a significant way. Without sexual desire there is not much opportunity for arousal to occur because initiation of sexual activity often does not progress to that point. It was found that the use of Viagra is quite limited in situations with underlying psychological or relationship problems (Berman, Berman, & Bumiller, 2001).

Pfizer's clinical trials with Viagra targeted women with physiological arousal disorder as the most prominent feature of their sexual dysfunction. The list of excluding criteria contained, among others, primary female orgasmic disorder, hypoactive sexual desire disorder, and potentially confounding medical and/or psychosexual problems. Concerning hypoactive sexual desire disorder, the screening instructions to the investigators stated in particular that even if a woman does not initiate sexual activity but in the process becomes responsive and aroused once sexual activity is started, the woman should be excluded for trial purposes.

Making hypoactive sexual desire one of the exclusionary criteria resulted in a low number of women eligible for inclusion into the clinical trials at some of the trial sites. Furthermore, as the double-blind, randomized, placebo-controlled trial proceeded, participants treated with sildenafil at doses of 10 mg, 50 mg, and 100 mg did not demonstrate improvement on any measure of sexual function beyond that achieved in placebo-treated women (Basson, McInnes, Smith, Hodgson, & Koppiker, 2002).

Pharmaceutical Investigations: Testosterone

On the pharmaceutical side, testosterone supplementation in individuals with testosterone levels below the normal range seems to be the treatment of choice. Authors such as Jennifer Berman and Laura Berman (2001) discuss testosterone as the hormone that affects sexual desire and mention that studies have shown that testosterone improves sexual desire and response.

Intramuscular Estrogen-Androgen Application

In one of the early studies on estrogen effects (Sherwin & Gelfand, 1987), 43 women who had undergone hysterectomy with oophorectomy were randomized to receive monthly intramuscular administration of either an estrogen, an estrogen-androgen combination, or a control preparation for a period of 8 months. In the group of women receiving the combination estrogen-androgen therapy, significantly increased sexual desire, frequency of sexual fantasies, and sexual arousal were reported compared to women in the estrogen-only and control groups. It was found, however, that the levels of estrogen and testosterone obtained from the women in the study exceeded the normal female range.

In a long-term study on the effects of androgens on increased bone mineral density and improved libido, 34 naturally or surgically postmenopausal women were randomized to receive either subcutaneous estrogen or combination estrogen plus testosterone implants (Davis, McCloud, Strauss, & Burger, 1995). The implants were administered every 3 months for 2 years. Significant increases in libido, activity, satisfaction, and pleasure were reported for the women who received the combination estrogen-testosterone therapy compared to the estrogen-only therapy.

Oral Application Of Estrogen-Testosterone Combinations

In a small study with 20 naturally or surgically postmenopausal women who were dissatisfied with estrogen monotherapy participants were randomly assigned to receive either oral esterified estrogen or combined esterified estrogen plus methyltestosterone for 4 weeks (Sarrel, Dobay, & Wiita, 1998). Significantly improved sexual desire and satisfaction as well as increased frequency of intercourse were reported for the combined estrogen-methyltestosterone therapy group. The estrogen-only therapy reportedly had no effect.

There are some potential concerns about the use of testosterone in women, such as virilization (hirsutism, acne, voice deepening, alopecia), which seem to be dose-related and not associated with all routes of administration. Liver toxicity and decreases in high-density lipoprotein may be associated with oral-substituted testosterones; transdermal or subcutaneous administration does not seem to be linked to adverse effects (Lobo, Rosen, Yang, Block, & Van Der Hoop, 2003).

Transdermal Patch: "Intrinsa"

Because many surgically menopausal women experience decreased sexual desire and pleasure as well as a decreased general sense of well-being despite estrogen therapy, Procter & Gamble Pharmaceuticals funded a series of studies focusing on this problem. Shifren and colleagues (2000) investigated the effects of transdermal testosterone replacement on sexual dysfunction in surgically menopausal women receiving estrogen-replacement therapy (ERT). The design was based on a double-blind, randomized, placebo-controlled crossover study including three treatment periods (Screen/Baseline—4 weeks; Periods I, II, and III—12 weeks each).

The study included women between the ages of 20 and 55 years who had undergone surgical menopause within a time period of 1 to 10 years prior to the study. They had to be in a stable, monogamous, heterosexual relationship for more than 1 year; they had to feel less satisfied with their sex life since the surgery and be desirous of improvement. Excluded from the study were women who had experienced more than 20 moderate-to-severe hot flashes per week while on ERT, who had used androgens during the past 3 months, or who had ongoing psychiatric disturbances or physical limitations affecting sexual function. During the study, all participants were maintained on an oral-conjugated equine estrogens (CEE) dose (≥ 0.625 mg/day) with twice weekly application of placebo or testosterone patches. Participants received either two placebo patches, or one testosterone and one placebo patch, or two testosterone patches.

To assess sexual function, a 22-item self-report questionnaire, the Brief Index of Sexual Function in Women (BISF-W), was used. The questionnaire tapped seven dimensions, such as thoughts of sexual activity and desire, sexual arousal, frequency of sexual activities, receptivity or initiation of sexual activities, orgasm and pleasure, relationship satisfaction, and problems related to sexual activity. In addition, 28-day telephone-based diaries were obtained along with adverse event assessments. The beginning sample of 75 women was reduced to 57 women in Period III with a mean age of 47 years and a mean time since surgical menopause (oophorectomy and hysterectomy) of 4.7 years. Eighty-three percent of the women were Caucasian, 11% African American, 5% Hispanic, and 1% Asian.

The reported results for sexual activities occurring at least once per week as mentioned on the BISF-W for fantasies showed a significant increase for those participants in the 150-µg and 300-µg treatment groups over those who received placebos only. For masturbation activities, increases over placebo were equal for the two different treatment groups (150 µg versus 300 µg), indicating that the higher dose did not have a stronger effect on frequency of masturbation than the lower dose. But for actual intercourse frequency the effects of the 150-µg dose were apparently the same as those of the placebo—although both were significantly elevated over baseline—and only the 300-µg dose yielded a higher-than-placebo frequency. This would indicate that the placebo served as well as the administration of the lower dose to focus the women's attention to some degree on sexual activities, but only the higher dose actually created an increase in sexual interest due to the medication.

The investigators chose to discuss their findings in terms of significantly increased frequency of sexual activity, orgasms, and psychological well-being at the higher testosterone dose. The treatment was well tolerated locally and systematically without clinically significant effects on hirsutism, acne, cholesterol, glucose, or insulin levels. Free and bioavailable testosterone levels showed increases in dose-dependent manner within physiologic range. Estrogen concentrations did not show changes.

Two Phase II clinical studies were conducted: Braunstein and colleagues (2003) reported on a study investigating the safety and efficacy of three doses of transdermal testosterone in surgically menopausal women with hypoactive sexual desire disorder (HSDD). The treatment population consisted of 447 surgically menopausal women receiving oral estrogen enrolled in a 24-week, randomized, double-blind, multicenter trial. The women received placebo (PL), or testosterone (T) 150, 300, or 450 μg by patch twice a week. Measures of frequency of satisfying sexual activity were obtained from responses to the sexual desire domain of the Profile of Female Sexual Function (PFSF) and records in the Sexual Activity Log (SAL).

The results at 24 weeks showed a 30% increase in frequency of total satisfying sexual activity in the 300 μg per day group as compared to the placebo group and an 81% increase when compared with baseline measures. Thus, the administration of 300 μg per day resulted not only in an increase in sexual activity compared to the beginning of the study but also a significant increase over the effects in the placebo group.

As in the earlier study, the 150 μg per day group was similar to the placebo group in frequency of satisfying sexual activity. The 450 μg per day group did not show an advantage over the 300 μg per day group, but an increase in hirsutism was reported (Simon et al., 2003). Dose-related increases in mean concentrations of total, free, and bioavailable testosterone were noted. The investigators stated that the androgen concentrations were significantly correlated with measures on the PFSF and SAL domains and concluded that in the Phase II study it was shown that the testosterone patch with the optimal dose of 300 μg per day improved sexual functioning and desire in oophorectomized women with HSDD.

Although a 150-μg testosterone patch will raise serum testosterone levels to that found in young females, it does not improve sexual function in oophorectomized women. Only the higher (300 μg) dose testosterone patch, which actually increases testosterone to physiologic levels above those that sustain sexual function in younger women, brought an improvement in sexual function for the oophorectomized women. According to Spark (2005), "Why women with HSDD require testosterone levels greater than they had when they were young to experience an improvement in sexual function has not yet been explained" (p. 284). Perhaps this is another indication and a reminder that there are other variables beside the levels of testosterone influencing women's sexual desire; psychological factors such as quality of the relationship or novelty of stimuli may have a stronger impact than is generally expected. Of the Phase II participants, 155 women agreed to continue in a 6-month safety extension. They were randomized to receive placebo or a 300 μg per day transdermal testosterone patch (Simon et al., 2002). Safety assessments, including liver function, hematology, lipid profiles, carbohydrate metabolism, clotting parameters, hirsutism, and acne, showed no significant changes from baseline (Simon et al., 2003).

According to materials provided by representatives of Procter & Gamble, Phase III clinical trials (Investigation of Natural Testosterone In Menopausal Women (INTIMATE) SM 1 involving 562 women and INTIMATE SM 2 involving 533 women) observed surgically menopausal women with HSDD on stable doses of oral or transdermal estrogen in two 24-week, randomized, double-blind, multicenter groups. The participants were randomly assigned to either placebo or treatment with 300 µg per day groups. The mean age for both groups was 49 years; mean relationship time was 19 and 18 years, respectively; and the mean time since oophorectomy was 8.5 and 9.0 years.

Instruments used to obtain measures of treatment effects included the Sexual Activity Log (SAL), a weekly diary that reports intercourse and non-intercourse activity as well as the number of orgasms experienced; the Profile of Female Sexual Function (PFSF), a 30-day recall measuring several domains of sexual function, such as desire, pleasure, arousal, responsiveness, self-image, orgasm, and sexual concerns; and the Personal Distress Scale (PDS), another 30-day recall, measuring distress related to lack of interest in sex.

Data from the SAL showed a 74% increase in total satisfying sexual activity for the treatment group in INTIMATE SM 1 over baseline compared to a 33% increase in the placebo group. INTIMATE SM 2 showed a 51% increase for the treatment population compared to a 23% increase in the placebo group. The PFSF showed an increase in desire of 56% in the treatment group compared to 29% in the placebo group in INTIMATE SM 1; and INTIMATE SM 2 showed a 49% increase for the treatment group versus 18% for placebo groups. Improvements in all domains of the PFSF and PDS were statistically significant at the 0.05 level.

Significant improvement in all 7 domains of sexual functioning, including sexual desire, pleasure, arousal, orgasm, concerns, responsiveness, and self-image (as measured by the Profile of Female Sexual Function) were reported in the testosterone-patch group (Buster et al., 2005).

When looking at the time to observe effects of the treatment, it appeared that statistically significant increases in satisfying sexual activity began at weeks 5 to 8 and were maintained through weeks 21 to 24. Statistically significant increases in sexual desire were observed at weeks 4, 12, and 24. Statistically significant decreases in personal distress were observed at weeks 4, 8, 12, and 24. For all three criteria, the maximal effect was seen by 12 weeks and was maintained through the end of the study. Adverse events reported were similar for the testosterone patch and the placebo groups and included complaints of application site reaction, upper respiratory infection, headache, and hirsutism. However, there were no clinically significant changes in laboratory assessments in the two groups.

Because the majority of women enrolled in this study were Caucasian, fewer data are available regarding the treatment effects on patients of other racial backgrounds. All participants included in the study were surgically postmenopausal women receiving concomitant estrogen therapy; therefore, to evaluate the effects in naturally menopausal women additional studies will be needed. As the Women's Health Initiative study (Rossouw et al., 2002) raised concerns with long-term safety of estrogen and progestin therapy, this study evaluated short-term use, 24 weeks, of the transdermal testosterone patch treatment (Simon et al., 2005).

Other Testosterone Products

Although the FDA's rejection of the testosterone patch blocked the development of the first drug designed to treat women's sexual difficulties, U.S. physicians apparently prescribe the hormone "off-label"—without special approval—to women with hypoactive sexual desire disorder (Enserink, 2005).

Giving women testosterone formulations originally developed for use in men may introduce unclear dosing requirements. Imprecise methods, such as pill cutting, may be required for administration of an appropriate dose. This could result in excessive or inadequate testosterone levels. Also, inconsistent dosing, efficacy, and safety may be associated with compounded testosterone preparations available from specialty pharmacies that are not subject to rigorous quality control (Simon, 2005).

In addition to the transdermal testosterone patch discussed above, other testosterone products, such as lotion, gel, vaginal ring, and spray formulations, are in different phases of clinical development for the treatment of HSDD in women (Simon, 2005).

LibiGel

At the meeting of the International Society for the Study of Women's Sexual Health (ISSWSH) in Amsterdam on October 17, 2003, Antares Pharma, Inc., announced that BioSante, its U.S. licensee of LibiGel, a topical testosterone gel product, presented analysis of data of a U.S.-based, double-blind, placebo-controlled study. After 3 months of treatment, a 130% increase from baseline in the frequency of satisfying sexual events as measured by individual patient diaries was reported (Antares Pharma, 2003).

BioSante Pharmaceuticals commented on updated U.S. Food and Drug Administration (FDA) safety and efficacy guidance for the development of testosterone products for the treatment of female hypoactive sexual desire disorder, which had been announced on October 29, 2005, at the ISSWSH Annual Meeting in Las Vegas. Stephen M. Simes, president and chief executive officer of BioSante, was pleased that the FDA validated testosterone's potential as an effective therapy for HSDD and announced BioSante's plan on filing Phase III efficacy and safety protocols for their studies of LibiGel™, the company's testosterone gel.

According to BioSante, LibiGel is a formulation of bioidentical testosterone, which is applied one time daily on the arm or shoulder and is quickly absorbed through the skin, delivering testosterone evenly to the bloodstream in a noninvasive manner. It has been reported that in a Phase II clinical trial, LibiGel increased the number of successful and satisfying sexual events by 238%.

Compared to baseline and placebo this increase is statistically significant (Business Wire, 2005).

Other products reportedly are in varying phases of development, such as the testosterone gel Tostrelle (Cellegy); a testosterone vaginal gel (Columbia Labs); a testosterone cream, Androsorb (Novavax); and a measured-dose testosterone nasal spray Vivus (Vliet, 2005). There have also been reports about the possibility of Noven Pharmaceuticals and Procter and Gamble's developing a combined product, a testosterone-estradiol transdermal patch. Noven Pharmaceuticals is the maker of Vivelle DOT, an estradiol patch, and the Combi Patch, an estradiol-progestin patch (Vliet).

Lobo and colleagues (2005) pointed out that the effects of testosterone monotherapy are not known because the testosterone trials conducted so far involved women who were administered concomitant estrogen. They concluded that the etiology of HSDD is probably multifactorial, including both biological and psychological factors. Based on clinical and research data, Heiman (2002) raised the issue that the "hypoactive sexual desire category would be best subdivided into logical subcategories by age and hormonal status, as well as the DSM-IV modifiers of Lifelong/Acquired and Global/Situational" (p. 78).

Applying Findings to Practice

Oral administration of testosterone in lozenge form is a convenient way to boost a woman's feelings of general well-being in addition to facilitating an interest in sexual activities. When Lois, a young, surgically menopausal woman, sought help at a clinic for sexual dysfunction, blood tests revealed that her level of free testosterone was well below the normal range. Supplemental hormone administration seemed to perform miracles: Lois, although just as busy with her career, exercising, and household chores as ever, found time and energy for sex. Her husband was overjoyed and she felt pleased and confident in herself.

Lisa, a slim, attractive, non-menopausal woman in her early thirties complained of low sexual desire. Lisa's history revealed that she had always been extremely critical of herself, especially of her appearance. No matter how much she dieted, she was never slim enough to be satisfied with her looks. She continuously complained about her weight and being too fat, seeking validation from her husband, only again to point to her imperfections. Lisa's exaggerated concentration on her weight did not permit sexual enjoyment, which is not surprising.

In Lisa's case, once sexual activities started, she was able to become aroused and experience orgasm, but soon after completion of the sex act her self-criticism resurfaced and squelched any thoughts of wanting to engage again in activities that would reveal her body. Lisa's husband grew tired of constantly validating her only to be faced by her contradictions. He also resented the long periods between sexual activities and Lisa's lack of enjoyment in it. Blood tests revealed significantly lower-than-normal testosterone levels in her case too, and, once she was supplied with additional hormones, Lisa was able to forget for the moment her exaggerated worries about her body. She enjoyed sexual activities with her husband to the point of initiating sex. Another success story?

On her next visit with the physician Lisa was told that her recent blood tests had shown testosterone levels still way below the normal range, yet she had felt an increase in sexual desire. What accounted for the change? She explained it with an attitude change. The attitude change took time and a lot of effort, as will be described later in Chapter 10.

In the meantime, Lois experienced a reduction in her level of energy as well as in her sexual interest. Convinced that her testosterone levels had dipped significantly, she approached her physician for another prescription. Blood tests revealed that, indeed, her testosterone level was somewhat lower; however, it was still well within the normal range and the physician did not consider an increase in the dosage as appropriate. Lois was disappointed and angry about the physician's refusal to increase her dosage. As her energy and libido level continued to slip gradually, she looked for other treatment sources.

Sue's sexual interest had completely vanished. With two children to raise, she worked full-time, and attended college with the hope of landing a more stimulating and well-paying job; and so her energy level was low. Her husband helped with the children and household chores as much as he could. Sue loved her husband and felt guilty over not wanting to have sex with him. She finally sought help at a clinic for sexual dysfunction. Her blood test revealed an extremely low level of free testosterone. She received different types of testosterone supplement treatment; injections seemed to work best for her.

For about 3 months, Sue's sexual desire soared even though her activity level was as high as before. Several times she initiated sexual activities to the happy surprise of her husband. But it did not last; after those 3 months her testosterone levels dropped and her sex drive disappeared. Repeated blood tests showed that although not as high as it had been at the peak of her libido increase, her testosterone level was still within the normal range. Like Lois, Sue was disappointed when she heard that the physician was not willing to increase the treatment levels. "For men there is Viagra and Cialis and Levitra to help them with their sexual performance, but nobody cares enough about women to come up with real help," she stated sadly.

Objectively speaking, a woman's testosterone level may still be significantly above what it had been prior to treatment, but the change in her feelings from the peak level down to a somewhat lower level often results in an emotional reaction that is difficult to adapt to. Unfortunately, while under the beneficial impact of the elevated hormone, it is unlikely that a woman will make great changes in her lifestyle. Most likely, she will use this boost of energy and good feelings to continue to fulfill the demands of her busy life, gratefully adding sex to her schedule. It would be highly advantageous if during the period of the testosterone boost the woman could be persuaded to modify her attitudes about her sexual involvement and to reconstruct her lifestyle accordingly. In other words, a pharmaceutical treatment approach should be combined with a psychological approach to increase the potential for success.

As pointed out earlier, in many cases of long-standing lack of sexual desire, women have come to regard sex as one more chore to perform for others, namely, their husbands. Sex has long ceased to be an activity they consider engaging in for their own enjoyment. Because women are poorly trained to consider their own pleasure as a priority, they are not easily persuaded to do so. The focus on their own enjoyment is too often followed by guilt feelings. The experience of these feelings of guilt and remorse is a hard price to pay for a little enjoyment—better not even to think about it.

Pheromones: Hope or Hype?

Much time and effort have been invested in the study of pheromones, substances excreted by an animal and received by another animal of the same species that bring about behavioral or physiological responses related to the recipient's reproductive potential. Research has been reported about the synchrony effects on women's menstrual cycle when underarm essences from one woman were applied to the skin under the nose in other women (Russell, Switz, & Thompson, 1980), and the timing of ovulation could be influenced by applying extracts of preovulatory or postovulatory sweat essences (Stern & McClintock, 1998). Other studies have demonstrated the impact of male pheromones upon female physiology. Regular intercourse, genital stimulation in the presence of a man, or sleeping next to a male partner seemed to increase the incidence of fertile cycles in women (Burleson, Gregory, & Trevathan, 1991), resulted in higher levels of postovulatory estrogen (Cutler, Garcia, Huggins, & Preti, 1986) and perimenopausal estrogen (Cutler, Davidson, & McCoy, 1983), and even delayed onset of menopause (Leidy-Sievert, Waddle, & Canali, 2001; McCoy, Cutler, & Davidson, 1985).

Additionally, post hoc observations of a placebo-controlled trial of 20 recipients seemed to indicate that odorless underarm-sweat extracts from sexually active women brought about an increase in the likelihood that the female recipients would engage in sexual intercourse at least once per week (Cutler, 1987). This effect was reported by 73% of the pheromone users as compared with 11% of placebo users.

These and other studies have brought about the notion of developing synthetic versions of male and female human sex pheromones, odorless cosmetic additives which can be mixed with an alcohol-based fragrance, such as perfumes (Cutler & Genovese-Stone, 2000). Studies have been conducted in both men and women investigating whether pheromone use was influencing individuals' sociosexual behaviors, such as sexual intercourse, sleeping next to a romantic partner, petting, kissing, informal dating, formal dating, and self-stimulation. For the men using the pheromone, an increase in the frequency of sexual intercourse and of sleeping next to a romantic partner, as well as increases in petting, kissing, and affectionate behaviors were reported when compared to men using a placebo-spiked fragrance. Similarly, the sample of reproductive-aged women using the female pheromone reported increases in the frequency of sexual intercourse, sleeping next to a romantic partner, petting, kissing, and affectionate behaviors when compared to women in the placebo group. Neither men nor women in the pheromone-testing groups reported a significant increase in masturbation. The authors (McCoy & Pitino, 2002; Cutler, Friedmann, & McCoy, 1998) interpreted this finding to indicate that pheromones did not result in increased sexual motivation but increased sexual attractiveness.

Whether a presumed human sex-attractant pheromone could influence specific sociosexual behaviors of postmenopausal women was a question other investigators (Rako & Friebely, 2004) attempted to answer by partly replicating the McCoy and Pitino (2002) study. Data obtained from 44 women with an average age of 57 years and having experienced their final menstrual period 7 years ago were analyzed with regard to the sociosexual behaviors of frequency of sexual intercourse, sleeping next to a romantic partner, petting, kissing, and affection as a result of pheromone use. Each woman used her preferred fragrance with the pheromone-like additive. It was found that the frequency of petting, kissing, and affectionate behaviors increased significantly for the pheromone-use group when compared with placebo users. Increases in sexual intercourse and sleeping next to a romantic partner were not statistically significant in comparison to the placebo users.

The investigators reported an interesting observation: There seemed to be a trend toward an increased incidence of self-stimulation among the placebo users in the postmenopausal women involved in the study. However, no obvious explanation for the reported increase in masturbation by the control group participants was offered. Based on the research literature, what might have appeared to have the potential for a desire-increasing function, based on some of the findings (Cutler, 1987), has not been shown to produce conclusive results.

There are so many factors contributing to the complexity of women's sexual desire. The next Chapter will discuss explorations of biological, ethological, social, and psychological aspects of life in search of explanations for the sexual difficulties reported by women.

3
Bio-Ethological and Social-Psychological Explanations

Thinking about sexual desire as a biological force would equate it with other biological drives, such as hunger or thirst, which are regulated by the drive to avoid pain and seek pleasure. And one would assume that, as a biological drive, sexual desire would operate relatively steadily throughout the lifespan. Indeed, some researchers have found that older adults continue to be interested in sex as long as poor health does not affect their sexual desire; and women, in particular, do not seem to be affected in their sexual desire by aging (Masters, Johnson, & Kolodny, 1994). Others, however, (McKinlay & Feldman, 1994) have observed that sexual desire and frequency of sexual thoughts decrease with age for both men and women.

Biological Factors: Unequal Sex Drives?

Public opinion seems to assume and accept that, in general, women's sexual drive is not as strong as that of men. Perhaps based on observations of the link between testosterone and sexual desire in both men and women, combined with the observations of men's generally higher levels and the decline in physiological circulating androgen levels in women starting in their mid-20s, most people would consider lower sex drives in women to be a result of biological factors. In reproductive-aged women, the mean circulating testosterone levels decline with increasing age, so that a 40-year old woman would have a testosterone level of about half of that of a woman aged 21 (Zumoff, Strain, Miller, & Rosner, 1995).

Additionally, evolutionary theory provides a framework for focusing on the reproductive potential and reproductive investment of members of the opposite sex. Reproductive potential refers to the genetic and other resources that are passed on to offspring, whereas reproductive investment can be seen as the actual use of these resources for the well-being of the offspring (Geary, Vigil, & Byrd-Craven, 2004). The rate of reproduction is determined by the biological limit on how many offspring males and females can produce. For females the biological limit is marked by periods of time, such as gestation time, the length of postpartum nursing (which constitute high levels of parental investment), and finally menopause, which generally marks the end of the female's reproductive potential.

Even when she is not pregnant or nursing, opportunities for conception are further regulated by a woman's monthly cycle, during which ovulation occupies just a small window. For males, the reproductive limit is dependent on the number of sexually accessible females he can compete for. Although sexual accessibility for procreation is influenced by biological factors, the absence or presence of sexual desire can have an additional impact on sexual accessibility.

Considering women's reproductive biology, the occurrence of ovulatory shifts in female sexual desire has been regarded as an evolutional adaptation. Pillsworth and colleagues (2004) hypothesized that as conception probability increases sexual desire increases in women who are in committed long-term relationships. A second hypothesis stated that depending on a woman's evaluation of her primary partner's qualities, the shift in the woman's desire for the primary partner—compared with extra-pair partners—will increase as ovulation approaches.

Testing their hypotheses in a study involving 173 women who were not using oral contraceptives, the investigators found an ovulatory peak in sexual desire in the mated women, whereas for unmated women, sexual desire and conception probability were uncorrelated. Among the mated women, a higher level of conception probability seemed to coexist with higher levels of in-pair sexual desire compared with extra-pair desires. However, there was a significant interaction between length of relationship and level of desire; women in longer relationships tended to experience more desire for extra-pair partners during periods of high conception probability.

Psychological and Social Considerations

Some writers are concerned that women—to enhance their sexual desire—would be tempted to use drugs, such as patches, pills, gels, and nasal sprays to treat what are really social or psychological problems and could be more effectively dealt with psychological interventions and education (Enserink, 2005).

Depression and Low Sexual Desire

For women with low sexual desire who also suffer from depression, a logical first step would be to alleviate the depression. But, as mentioned in Chapter 1, the use of some antidepressant medication may result in lowering levels of libido. Mixed results were obtained in clinical trials of fluoxetine therapy (Michelson, Schmidt, Lee, & Tepner, 2001). At the start of their Phase I clinical trial, 73.9% of the women reported minimal to severe difficulties with low sexual desire prior to the beginning of the fluoxetine therapy. At the start of Phase II the proportion of women reporting low sexual interest had dropped to 50.3%. At the end of Phase II, 26.4% of the women reported improved, 47.3% unchanged, and 26.3% worsened sexual interest.

Considering this and other studies mentioned earlier, more research is needed to separate the effect of depression on sexual desire from the effect of antidepressants and to improve our understanding of the interaction among the conditions of depression and sexual desire and the exposure to antidepressant agents (West, Vinikoor, & Zolnoun, 2004).

In agreement with Lobo et al. (2005, mentioned in Chapter 2), Kingsberg (2005) pointed out that psychological and social factors as well as a woman's health status contribute to her sexual function. In fact, they may be more important than ovarian function as a woman ages. The partner relationship, previous level of pleasure from sexual activity, and mental and physical health are all factors impacting women's sexual interest and activities.

Studies of female sexual function typically include parameters such as satisfaction with the current sexual relationship, sexual desire, frequency of sexual intercourse, level of arousal, difficulty achieving orgasm, and pain during sex. Measures of sexual desire include sexual thoughts, fantasies, and dreams. Linking the concept of desire to Levine's (1992) "biopsychosocial" definition of desire and its three components—drive; personal beliefs, values, and expectations; and motivation, Kingsberg (2005) described drive as the biological, hormonal component which is experienced as spontaneous sexual interest and genital tingling accompanying sexual thoughts or fantasies.

In Kingsberg's (2005) view, drive is seen as the body's signal "that it would like to be sexual" (p. 4). Personal values and beliefs constitute the cognitive component of desire, influencing an increase or decrease of a woman's sexual interest. The psychological and interpersonal factors that persuade the woman to share her body with a partner in a sexual experience constitute the third component, motivation. Kingsberg suggested that clinicians who want to help patients with sexual dysfunction need to understand the concepts of desire and its subcomponents.

As an alternative view to the assumption that desire always precedes arousal, which, in turn, precedes orgasm, Basson (2001) proposed a different model. In some instances, women may start from a point of sexual neutrality. Seduction from the partner or the women's conscious decision to have sex may lead to arousal, which may then be followed by desire.

The myriad of factors impacting upon women's sexuality cannot be fully and completely covered within the confines of this book; however, mentioning some of them gives us an appreciation of the complexity involved when we attempt to understand women's sexual interests and sexual activities as we explore in more detail different aspects of women's sexual attitudes and behaviors.

The Oxytocinergic System's Link With Behavior and the Sexual Response

The etiology of differing sexual desire as resulting from combinations of biological factors in the oxytocinergic system was explored by several researchers (Anderson-Hunt & Dennerstein, 1995; Carter, 1992; Insel, 1997; Kaplan, 1995;

Leckman et al., 1994; Leedes, 1999). According to these researchers oxytocin (OT) is involved in every phase of the human sexual response. It is instrumental in the phenomenological experience of comfort/discomfort (e.g., comfort, anxiety, or avoidance) toward both sexual expression and interpersonal relating. In part, it is also responsible for the initiation and maintenance of sexually obsessive-compulsive behaviors. It has been hypothesized that once the nature of a person's sexual desire has been established (feelings of comfort or discomfort toward interpersonal attachments and toward erotic fantasies), the oxytocinergic system serves to maintain it rigidly because of oxytocin's relationship with both obsessive-compulsive behavior and the human sexual response.

Data from both animal and human studies suggest that minimal levels of OT may be linked to sexually avoidant behaviors, whereas increased levels of OT seem to occur in response to genital and/or genital tract stimulation and nipple aureole manipulation (Anderson-Hunt & Dennerstein, 1995). OT may also be released as a result of a conditioned response in the absence of direct stimulation. During certain stages of the developmental process, such as courtship periods, gestation and early mothering periods, organisms seem to be vulnerable for the development of obsessive compulsive behaviors, experiencing the urge to perform actions according to rigidly applied rules (Leckman et al., 1994). Disparate releases of OT mediate different emotional dispositions, which, in turn, account for varied forms of obsessive compulsive behaviors (Leedes, 1999).

Functional Aspects: "Love Maps"

Considering functional theories, the concept of sexual desire can be deconstructed into two conceptually meaningful variables that make up a person's love map. There may be an emotional disposition toward fantasy and an emotional disposition toward interpersonal relationships (Leedes, 1999). The term "love map" was originally conceptualized by Money (1986) as " ... a developmental representation or template in the ... brain depicting the idealized lover and the idealized program of sexuoerotic activity projected in imagery ..." (p. 20). These representations (love maps) are believed to begin to emerge by 3 to 5 years of age with mental imageries such as dreams and fantasies. According to Money, the love maps are "ineradicable."

The Concept of "Antifantasies"

On a functional basis, the nature of sexual desire has been described by several researchers in terms of being either relational or arelational (Kaplan, 1995; Leiblum & Rosen, 1988, 1989; Rosen & Leiblum, 1995). In Kaplan's view, arelational internal representations, such as fantasies, can up- or down-regulate individuals' sexual desire. Based on positive relational representations and negative relational representations toward other persons, disparate sexual motivational states are evoked at different times within the same individual. The concept of antifantasies was used by Kaplan to describe negative relational representations. Antifantasies are fearful or repugnant imaginings formed by individuals about prospective sexual partners. These antifantasies function to reduce or eliminate feelings of sexual expressiveness in the context of erotic or loving relationships.

Relational Aspects of Sexual Desire

Some regard sexual desire as a cognitive or emotional experience, such as a longing (Everaerd, 1988), while conceptualizing desire as one factor in a larger relational context emphasizes the relational aspects of sexual desire. The notion of sexual desire as a cognitive-emotional force considers it as originating within the individual, but others (Verhulst & Heiman, 1979) regard it as something that is outside the individual, such as an external stimulation from the desired object or person.

When sexual desire is conceptualized as either relational or arelational, the component of sexual desire which is arelational is internally represented by objectified or idealized fantasies, whereas the component of relational sexual desire is internally represented by Bowlby's (1973, 1980, 1988) concept of internal representations or Internal Work Models (IWMs), which, in part, project the degree of responsiveness of an attachment relationship. According to Bowlby (1973), "... the model of the attachment figure and the model of the self are likely to develop so as to be complementary and mutually confirming" (p. 238).

In childhood, the individual develops beliefs about the self that are regulated by the perceived responsiveness of the primary caregiver. Usually the primary caregiver serves as an expectant model for future close relationships and is also instrumental in the individual's formulating beliefs about the self: i.e., "I am (un) worthy of consistent care." According to Bowlby (1988) the desire for a secure attachment or "a secure base," which provides responsiveness and affirmation, is the prototypical "older desire." Within a profusion of sexually diverse symbols, the subject is able to glory in the responsiveness and affirmation dispensed by the object.

In this conceptual framework, sexual desire can be interpreted as a yearning for a projected affectionate and bonding primal experience to which the individual would ideally respond in kind. The experience may develop on either a humanistic and relational, or objectified and arelational basis. Sexual desire is expressed by both types of internal representations, the ones that depict comfortable interpersonal relationships and the ones that constitute objectified/idealized fantasies, which depict comfort through metaphors, providing an imagined responsiveness by the object and an imagined worthiness toward the subject.

As metaphoric reflections of interpersonal relationships, fantasies serve to mediate the nature of sexual desire in people. Individuals who have an emotional predisposition toward discomfort with interpersonal relationships have a greater tendency to fantasize than persons who have a love map characterized by an emotional disposition ("personal bias") of comfort with interpersonal relationships.

Relationships lacking in open communication often prevent the development of true emotional intimacy between the two partners. In the absence of intimacy, partners may have difficulty expressing their wishes and preferences during sexual activity. Not getting what one wants or not receiving feedback about one's ability to please one's partner often leads one or both partners to resort to fantasies in order to reach sexual gratification. One partner's sexual fantasy life may revolve about other individuals who are completely outside the relationship. In the erotic dreamworld some imaginary individual may be occupying the body of the uninformed other partner.

Social Constructionist Considerations

The increase in female sexuality brought on by the sexual revolution was seen as evidence by some that female sexuality in the past had been under the influence of social and cultural suppression (Baumeister & Twenge, 2002). However, a point to reflect on is that the sexual revolution, which had produced a greater change in female than in male sexuality, occurred during the second half of the 1960s through the 1970s and into the early 1980s, but today we are still—or again—concerned with the complaint of low libido in women. About 30% of all women at least until age 60 years are affected by lack of interest in sex (Baumeister & Twenge). One might be tempted to ask, "Was the sexual revolution a transient phenomenon—perhaps a response or reaction to a different set of circumstances than commonly assumed?"

Considerations of a suppression theory raise the question, "Who is responsible for the suppression? Are suppression efforts exerted generally by men or by women themselves?" Baumeister and Twenge (2002) have attempted to explore that question because the answer leads to "competing predictions that men or women would be the main proximal sources of influence toward suppression of female sexuality" (p. 167).

Considering the case that suppression of female sexuality was instituted by men, the goal might have been to withhold sexual pleasure from women. The benefits of stifling female sexuality would be reaped mainly by husbands through assuring a wife's fidelity and eliminating paternity-related doubts. Feminists, on the other hand, would tend to interpret men's stifling of female sexuality as mechanisms of control and victimization (Travis & White, 2000).

Another line of argument holds that insatiable female sexuality would be threatening to men because of men's greater physical sexual limitations, such as men's refractory period and the visible nature of men's lack of arousal, and their inability to have multiple orgasms (Hyde & DeLamater, 1997). The arguments involving men's developing a system for the oppression of women's sexuality assume that women would want to engage in frequent sexual activities with multiple partners, which would produce chaos and undermine the social order. Thus, men, seeking to protect a social order that is to their benefit, have instituted a system of penalties and punishment for female sexual activities outside the marriage bed.

Sexuality and Social Exchange Considerations

In contrast to opinions pointing toward men's attempts to stifle women's sexual desire and expression, another theory suggests that women have taken an active part in suppressing female sexual desire. Arguments supporting this line of reasoning have cited social exchange theory, which analyzes human behavior in terms of costs and rewards. Starting with the assumption that sex is a resource possessed by women and wanted by men, men must offer women other desired resources (money, commitment, security, etc.) to obtain the desired commodity from the women (Baumeister & Tice, 2000). Insofar as the man desires a sexual relationship more than the woman, she is at an advantage and he has to provide other benefits that will persuade her to have sex with him.

According to this view, sex assumes the characteristics of an object for trade and limiting the availability of the commodity keeps the price that can be extracted from men high in terms of other resources. On the other hand, if sex were easily available from women in general, wives or girlfriends might be apprehensive about losing their men in a sexually competitive society. In order to maintain a high price for sexual interaction, women would have to act in agreement in restricting the availability of the resource. A provider of cheaper sex would thus become a threat to the rest of them and would expose herself to criticism and punishment.

Lists of arguments have been proposed in support of each gender's exerting control on female sexual drives, but much of the evidence seemed to lead to the conclusion that the proximal causes of the suppression of female sexuality are mostly female. Although institutional attempts to stifle female sexuality may be male in origin (courts, police, etc.), the agents carrying out the regulating or stifling efforts were mostly female (mothers influencing daughters' sexuality and being the main parental restraining influence on daughters' sexual behaviors; female peer groups helping members to keep from going too far sexually; women being more judgmental regarding other women's sexual indiscretions, or regarding prostitution, etc.). Could those female agents who were instrumental in suppressing women's sexuality perhaps be seen as identifying with the (male) oppressor, a concept proposed some time ago by Sigmund Freud?

Considering another study involving a sample of highly sexual women who reportedly desired sex at least seven times per week, similar attitudes were expressed when it was found that the women had experienced significant problems in their relationships with other women and had been subjected to pressure to reduce their sexual activity (Blumberg, 2000). The women stated that they felt much more comfortable and accepted by men than by women.

As some of the most significant evidence in support of the female suppression hypothesis, Baumeister and Twenge (2002) mention the drastic measures used in some non-Western cultures. Practices of genital surgery to curtail female sexuality are outlawed in Western countries but are still practiced in other parts of the world. Apparently, decisions regarding the surgery are made by the mothers or grandmothers of the girls and the operation itself is usually performed by a woman, such as a midwife. Furthermore, when men in those countries were questioned about these practices they seemed to indicate that they would prefer women whose sexuality had not been stifled by the surgical methods.

If the evidence significantly supports the female suppression hypothesis, what are the reasons for women to engage in stifling female sexuality? Are women suppressing each other's sexuality out of altruistic motives because of the risks connected with sexual activities, such as sexually transmitted diseases and unwanted pregnancies? Or is the goal to influence the sexual marketplace so that they can avoid having sex without being afraid that other women will supply it to their boyfriends or husbands? "Women might be tempted to think that if they band together and all refuse sex, men will have to acquiesce and learn to do without as much sex as they want. In particular, women may feel that they can be sexually unresponsive without risk of losing their male partners as long as the men cannot find other, more satisfying partners, and so suppressing other women's sexuality is vital" (Baumeister & Twenge, 2002, p. 199).

Malleability of Women's Sexuality

Reviewing many studies, Baumeister (2000) observed that women vary more than men in their sexuality. Their frequency of sexual activity may change depending on whether they are involved in a relationship. Another insight gained from the literature review was that women's sexual attitudes and behaviors did not seem as consistent as those associated with men's sexuality. As an example Baumeister pointed out that women, more so than men, have the tendency to engage in sex when they do not feel like it or not engage in sex even though they may feel like having sex. Based on these observations, Baumeister raised the question whether women's sexuality might be more malleable than men's in response to situational, cultural, or social conditions.

The answer may be found in considering that historically women's sexuality much more so than men's was shaped by cultural and social factors; in fact, men were generally a big part of those environmental conditions or constrictions. Not so long ago women found themselves in situations where they had to engage in sex whether they liked it or not as it was the husband's right, and where they had to make compromises about sex—and many still do in order to keep an intact marriage for the benefit of their children. In other words, out of necessity women adapt to the demands made on them by the environment.

Some support for the notion of women's greater sexual malleability or "erotic plasticity" reportedly comes from studies that investigated changes in women's sexual identity. For instance, in one study focusing on 18–25-year-old women who were identified as lesbian or bisexual (Diamond, 2003), apparently, one-fourth of these young women changed their sexual identity over a period of 5 years. Other researchers reported changes in women's sexual interests from heterosexual to a lesbian orientation (Kitzinger & Wilkinson, 1995) and from a lesbian to a bisexual or heterosexual identity (Bart, 1993; Rust, 1992).

Louise: Changing to Lesbian Relationship

Louise, a young divorced woman and mother of two children, realized that she was more comfortable living with another woman than with a man. Her marriage to a controlling husband had been extremely stressful to her. He demanded Louise's subservience in running and maintaining the family household and he expected her to be available for sex five to six times a week, which he needed for relief from his stressful job. If his demands were not fulfilled, he was not a gentle person. Often the sexual activity was accompanied by punches and blows to Louise's body. To protect her children, Louise complied as much as she could with her husband's demands until one day he did not only leave bruises but a few broken ribs. A friend took her to the emergency room, taking her children along too. After Louise received emergency care and her friend saw to it that the event was properly documented in the medical files, her friend brought Louise and her children to her own home and with the help of the friend's husband, arranged temporary quarters for them. The friend's husband also accompanied Louise to her home to pack some clothing for herself and the children.

In spite of the restraining order Louise had obtained against her husband, she and her children went through several months of torment and frequent moves to escape the wrath of the husband. It took 2 years for Louise to work through these problems to a point where she could give her life some stability. She found a job as server in a restaurant and entered a community college, which allowed her to work slowly on a career that would enable her to provide for herself and her children. About midway through her studies she became involved with another female student and they entered into a committed relationship.

Was her decision based on the disappointments lived through in her heterosexual relationship with her husband, or would she eventually have found her true sexual identity in a lesbian relationship even if her marriage had been happier? Had she experienced longings for another woman earlier in her life but chosen to get married because a lesbian lifestyle would not have been acceptable to her parents and friends and because she wanted to avoid the pain and struggle resulting from going against social and cultural norms?

Louise did not remember any strong sexual feelings for any of her girlfriends as she grew up, although she did enjoy their company. What she does recollect is a strong wish for motherhood. As an only child, raised by a single mother, she tried to mother the younger children in her neighborhood. Her goal for motherhood might have overshadowed any sexual feelings for girls if indeed she had experienced any. The wish for motherhood had kept her from pursuing a career. Louise admitted that after her divorce she tried to date a few men but did not feel she could trust them. Now she feels loving and comfortable in the relationship with her female partner.

In general, women are more likely to be influenced by the context in which sex occurs than men are (Williams, 1983). Negative qualities in the relationship or in the immediate situation tend to bother women more than men. Although it would not be correct to say men are not bothered by the quality of the relation-ship, for women, their sexual responsiveness may be more contingent on those qualities. Women often do not understand how their partners can be in the mood for making love after just having been involved in an argument with them. Women's hurt feelings seem to have a longer life in their memory, making it dif-ficult to respond in a loving way and influencing their overall sense of sexual satisfaction.

Sexual Satisfaction

The search for explanations concerning women's sexual desire is made compli-cated by the terminology used in the various studies on this subject. Not only is there a lack of clearly defined criteria when the word *desire* is used in the differ-ent studies, the use of the term "sexual satisfaction" adds to the complexity. Regan and Berscheid (1999) strongly recommended to differentiate clearly between sexual desire and sexual activity. And just as sexual activity does not always include sexual desire, sexual satisfaction may or may not include sexual desire. Engaging in sexual activity does not necessarily mean that sexual desire for the activity was experienced by all participants. Sexual satisfaction may mean the participant was satisfied with the sexual event, even though it may not have started with the experience of sexual desire.

A discussion of "The National Survey on Christian Female Sexuality" con-ducted by Debra Taylor, Archibald Hart, and Catherine Hart Weber stated that many Christian women report high levels of sexual satisfaction. A happy mar-riage, frequency of sexual intercourse, orgasm, and lovemaking sessions lasting from 30 to 60 minutes were factors associated with sexual satisfaction. According to the report, 30% of the respondents experienced greater satisfaction when their sexual activities occurred two to three times per week (Richard, 2000).

This frequency is somewhat higher than what had been reported for the general population in the 1994 University of Chicago study "Sex in America," and the principal investigator explained the higher rates with the desire by Christian women to please their mates, who prefer more frequent sex. This seems to echo one of the respondent's statements that satisfying her husband's needs was of greater importance than her own orgasm. But like women in the general popula-tion, Christian women also seemed to have difficulty with their energy level when it came to sex. Almost half of the respondents stated that having the energy for sex was their greatest difficulty, followed by feeling desire. Additionally, body image had an impact on Christian women's sexual satisfaction.

Thus, the above study seems to confirm that sexual activities can come about for many different reasons other than sexual desire itself. An individual can par-ticipate in sexual activities to please a partner, to express love, to fulfill a per-ceived obligation, or as result of having been coerced, situations that seem particularly relevant to females.

Hypersexual Behaviors, Sexual Addiction, or Sexual Compulsion?

Although general opinion accepts the notion of men's greater sex drive, there are also highly sexual women in existence. While many women may envy other women with high sexual desire, and men might say they would like to find them, the lives of highly sexed women are not as problem-free as many might assume. Growing up as a woman with high sexual interest in a society that almost denies this characteristic to women by ascribing it mostly to men can be a traumatic experience. Being different from the norm of young girls who are expected to become sexually awakened by the "right" man, may provoke self-doubt and low self-esteem in those who are confronted with their own sexuality. Furthermore, these women's intense sexuality may lead to strained relationships with other females, as mentioned in the Blumberg (2000) study above. It may even isolate them from other girls and women.

Problems of Highly Sexual Women

In an exploratory study involving 44 highly sexual women aged 20 to 82, participants were asked to describe their actual frequency of and preference for sexual activity, specifying sexual events, not orgasms (Blumberg, 2003). The term "highly sexual" was based on two descriptive categories: (1) women who desire sexual stimulation six to seven times per week or more and who act on that desire; and (2) women who regard themselves as highly sexual women and who have sex on their mind often; it is an aspect that strongly and frequently affects their behaviors.

As reported by the women, the internally sensed demand for sexual excitement was too strong to be ignored, and it affected their daily lives in organizing and scheduling their time and energies. The women reported how they had learned to make conscious decisions about their own identity and how to lead their lives. For many of them, this introspection had helped them to gain self-confidence. Others had felt for years that their sexuality was an affliction that needed to be repressed. Main negative themes in the women's reports included the struggle in finding and maintaining sexually satisfying relationships, a difficulty in relationships with other women, and a sense of not being understood or accepted by society.

The Difficulty of Achieving Sexual Satisfaction Within a Single Relationship

Another common theme that emerged was the difficulty the women experienced in trying to achieve sexual satisfaction within a single primary relationship. It seemed almost impossible to find a single man who could meet their needs. Almost every woman in this study admitted that at some time in her life she had sought out multiple partners to satisfy her sexual needs. More than 70% of the participants either were still involved with more than one sex partner or considered it an available option.

For some of the women in the study a situation of polyamory, a type of open marriage in which partners agree to have intimate and sexual relationships outside the primary relationship, might have been desirable. People who practice polyamory describe their arrangement as one of multiple loving, consensual relationships with an emphasis on emotional commitment—and quite distinguished from the concept of "swinging." Polyamory is conceived of as "responsible nonmonogamy," where more than two people are connected in an honest, ethical relationship (Graham, 1998). Unfortunately, the women in the above-mentioned study might not have found spouses that agreed with the concept of polyamory.

It is not surprising that many of the participants admitted that they had been labeled with terms historically used to pathologize the behaviors of sexually active women. The terms *nymphomania, applied to women, and—satyriasis* when applied to men—has been around for a long time, but more recently "sexual addiction" has been used to label compulsive sexual behavior. The investigator disagreed on two grounds with the use of these labels in connection with his study participants. He argued that according to some professionals (Levin, 1987) "addicts lose personal control over their behavior to the degree that they unpredictably engage in or ignore aspects of life necessary for daily functioning" (Blumberg, 2003, p. 153) and that addictive behavior is believed to increase in frequency or intensity over time and thereby will have increasing negative effects on the person's life. According to Blumberg, neither condition was met by the women in his study. The women in the study did not fit the criteria for compulsion nor for addiction.

However, the author believes that the information about the participants' arousal and desire provides "evidence of a biological substrate, one that can and does affect some women's lives strongly" (Blumberg, 2003, p. 154). On the other hand, the idea of a biological substrate does not eliminate the importance of the social construction and feminist analysis models of female sexuality development.

Cindy: Problematic Sex Drive

Cindy, a pretty redhead, had not experienced any traumatic events as she was growing up; neither had her cousin Ruth. Both girls became aware early on of their intense need for sexual stimulation and satisfaction. They called it the "family curse." Cindy was troubled by her sexual preoccupation which none of her girlfriends seem to share. Talking to Ruth helped to reduce the feelings of isolation; at least Cindy was not the only one with this affliction. It was Ruth who thought of a solution: they both needed to get married as soon as they could because they would have husbands who could then satisfy their needs legitimately, Ruth reasoned.

Cindy took Ruth's suggestion to heart; right out of high school she married Tom, the boy she had been dating. During their early years of marriage they were sexually very active even though Cindy gave birth to three daughters, with two of them being identical twins. The girls were still quite young when Tom lost his job. He had difficulty finding other employment and finally Cindy went to work as a cashier at a local supermarket. Tom began feeling sorry for himself. To pass the time he spent at home when other men were at work, he took up drinking. The alcohol did not have a positive effect on his personality. By the time Cindy returned from work he was usually too drunk to help her with any of the chores. When she criticized him, he resorted to beating her. Although Cindy still felt her intense sexual desire, she could not bear for Tom to touch her after the first severe beating.

Cindy realized that she was emotionally and sexually vulnerable to any man who showed her kindness. After her divorce Cindy was just as vulnerable but, at least, she did not have to worry about committing adultery. Unfortunately, her sexual needs made her an easy prey for men who wanted sex without commitment. She often felt taken advantage of but the physical closeness and the sexual excitement were propositions too seductive to resist. Some of the men she entered into an early sexual relationship with later held it against her and put her down for the pleasure that she had given them. They actually scolded her for the example she set for her daughters.

Cindy would have agreed with Rhesa, a young divorced mother who had been criticized by a male friend for being willing to start a sexual relationship with him. Rhesa stated, "It's really confusing; when I was a young girl, men tried to convince me that I was a sexual being—as they called it. Now that I am single again but have children, all I am supposed to be is a mother. I still long for the intimacy and fulfillment of a sexual relationship. Men don't seem to have the same problems" (Maass & Neely, 2000, p. 130).

Along with Cindy and Rhesa is Susie, an attractive, passionate woman with a strong sex drive. In almost 20 years of marriage she tried to keep passion and sexual intimacy in her relationship with Rick, her husband. Rick's opinion was that having sex once or twice a week was more than the average couple engaged in and that was plenty for him. He was neither curious nor adventurous and sex remained a weekly perfunctory event. Susie left the marriage when the children reached college age. Now she is on her own, starting her life over but has nobody to share it with and—except for masturbation—is having sex less than before. She is frustrated; she has so much to give and nobody is there to receive it.

Attachment/Abandonment Issues

The reasons for women to experience a greater desire for sex may be as varied as the reasons for those who feel less of a desire for sex. Some women may regard sex as a confirmation of their worth. Daily sexual intercourse may give them the feeling of security. They might reason that, as long as they are still being desired by their partners, their world is safe and their existence is not threatened by abandonment.

Beth: Sex for Security

Beth, a woman in her middle thirties and the mother of a little girl, is a sad example of this kind of reasoning process, using sex for confirmation and security. When Beth and Tim, her fourth husband, were referred to a clinic for sexual dysfunction, Tim was the identified client with the stated problem of low libido. Beth was attractive in a quiet type of way, with an air of vulnerability about her. People reached out to her and wanted to protect her.

Her vulnerability had originated in childhood when her parents divorced and her father moved away. The abandonment she experienced from her father's move was compounded by the series of stepfathers her mother introduced to her. None of her mother's marriages lasted more than 3 or 4 years. The only element of stability in this scenario was the string of replacements of father figures.

In an individual session with Tim, he admitted that his first impulse after seeing Beth was to take care of her. Her initial quietness seemed to promise gentle personality traits, just what Tim had looked for all his life. The fact that Beth had a little daughter from a previous marriage made the situation even more desirable; now he had two precious females to pamper and protect. The first several months of their marriage were a continuous honeymoon. Beth could hardly wait for him to come home to continue their passionate lovemaking that they usually started in the morning before leaving for work.

Then came times when Tim was not up to having sex in the morning because he wanted to sleep a little longer before getting up for work. Beth seemed disappointed but doubled her efforts at the end of the day. Tim realized that it was rare to have a quiet evening at home without sexual activity. Although many of his colleagues envied him, Tim felt more that he had to engage in sexual intercourse on a daily basis in order to preserve the peace in the family. On those occasions when Tim was not interested in sex, Beth's behavior became complaining, accusing, angry, and depressed. But the more he felt forced to have sex, the less he liked it.

When Beth related her side of the situation she expressed her suspicion that Tim might be interested in someone else. In response to the question about the reasons for her suspicion, she simply said, "if he does not want it with me, he must be getting it somewhere else." After three failed marriages, Beth did not have much faith in that type of commitment. The man's sexual desire for her seemed to be the only yardstick by which to measure her safety. As long as she fulfilled her man's sexual needs, she would not be abandoned as she had been in the past. This was a lesson she thought she had learned from her first marriage. If a man does not have strong and frequent sexual desire for his wife, the wife's security might be in jeopardy.

Her most important romantic relationship had been with Ben, a gentle and talented young man who seemed different from anyone she had known. Unlike other young men, Ben did not press her for sex. He seemed patient and understanding. Beth felt secure with him. But one night they did have sex and Beth found Ben to be a wonderful lover. For the next several months Beth thought she had the perfect relationship and her thoughts centered on marriage.

When she found out that she was pregnant she told Ben, hoping that he would be happy. But he seemed shocked rather than happy. Ben confessed that he was gay. He had hoped that his relationship with Beth would help him in overcoming his homosexual orientation. Beth was stunned. Ben explained that although he would be in favor of an abortion, he would marry her if she decided to have the baby. However, he added they would most likely divorce after a while. Beth rejected the idea of an abortion and hearing that Ben was willing to marry her sounded to her like a commitment for life.

During the 3 years of their marriage, sexual activities were rare. Beth's hopes for a change in Ben's sexual orientation were unsupported, and divorce was the inevitable outcome of Beth's romantic dreams. With her first and following marriages Beth learned that marriage was not a guarantee against abandonment. Because the sexual area had been the main problem in her first marriage, she regarded sex as the glue in all later relationships. As soon as the frequency of sexual intercourse fell below once a day, her fears surfaced and she usually expressed them with complaints and accusations.

Her complaining behavior only served to speed up the deterioration of the relationship she was in. As long as Beth was not able to find different measures and indications for a happy relationship, she was doomed to repeat her behavioral patterns, which sooner or later prompted the men to leave her. She was assured to get more of what she had been afraid of all along—being abandoned.

Most people would interpret Beth's use of the frequency of sexual intercourse as measure of her security as a sign of her self-doubt or low level of self-esteem. Individuals with low self-esteem look to others for their affirmation. Therefore, they look with high hopes to their partner, expecting assurance while at the same time fearing rejection once the partner gets to know their imperfections. The mixture of high expectations and anticipated disappointment and rejection places the individual on an emotional roller coaster where it is impossible to relax and enjoy the company of the partner. In some women, the initial sexual desire that came from the individual's high hopes for affirmation may dwindle under the onslaught of the anxiety.

Sexual Victimization and High Sex Drive

Several investigators have suggested that sexually very active women had been sexualized at an early age by incest or other inappropriate contacts with adults (Finkelhor & Browne, 1985; Meston, Heiman, & Trapnell, 1999; Westerlund, 1992). These hypotheses may be true for some cases where retrospective studies revealed that the women had been victims of incest or other inappropriate sexual contacts.

Liz: Sexually Insatiable?

Roger brought his wife Liz into therapy with the comment that Liz was sexually insatiable. He stated that she would like to engage in sex at least twice a day. At periods in their married life when Roger was not able to comply with her wishes, Liz had become involved in extramarital affairs.

As Liz, a rather plain-looking woman in her mid-30s, related her background history, she admitted that her father had sexually abused her when she was a child. In addition, he had encouraged her older brother to do the same as he demonstrated his version of what he considered "sex education." Liz was not beaten during the sexual abuse and made no mental or emotional connection to the concept of punishment or abuse. Her mother, an emotionally unavailable woman, apparently did not know or care about what was happening to Liz.

Later in high school, Liz was not one of the popular girls, mostly because of her plainness, but she was good-natured and thus was allowed to function on the periphery of the accepted group. Boys found her accessible for sex, and she earned a reputation for her fellatio skills. Because none of the boys dated her seriously, she remained on good terms with the girls in her group despite her sexual activity. The other girls did not see her as a threat. And Liz did not pose a threat to anybody; she enjoyed the attention she received for her sexual favors and developed a craving for it.

Although her craving for sexual attention was about to cost her her marriage, Liz did not blame her father who had died almost 10 years ago, for her "addiction," if we want to call it that. How did Liz resolve her situation? She slowly learned to re-focus her thoughts when she felt the urge for sex. In addition, she was able to schedule time for herself to treat her body to a leisurely bath, using plenty of lotion and perfume afterward, and masturbating.

Part of her training was to recognize her body as her own property that she could treat as nicely as she wanted without depending on the attention of others. As she spent more time on herself and improved her make-up skills, Liz actually became more attractive. With her improved self-esteem Liz considered entering college and applying for acceptance in a nursing program.

Was it the attention or the physical sensations of sex that Liz had come to crave? Her answer to this question was, "Both; it was difficult to distinguish where one left off and the other started. Now I have come to understand that both the attention and the physical sensation are very important to me. And I have finally found ways to get both without losing the love of my husband."

Sexual Addiction Versus Compulsion

There is disagreement among professionals as to whether the behavior of individuals with significantly elevated sexual desire may fall into the classification of "sexual addiction." The term was introduced by Patrick Carnes (1983, 1996) to make a connection between some atypical or paraphilic behaviors as outward symptoms manifesting a process of psychological addiction. Carnes drew similarities to the four phases of a typical addiction cycle. In the first phase, the individual is preoccupied with obsessive thoughts about a particular sex behavior. This *preoccupation* phase often includes certain *ritualistic* behaviors, which intensify the sexual excitement that started to build up in the preoccupation phase. The actual expression of the *sexual act* is often followed by *despair* when the individual is overwhelmed by feelings of depression and anxiety. As the cycle is repeated, the individual's depression is replaced by a sexual high, which is in some ways similar to the high achieved by mood-altering chemicals such as alcohol or cocaine.

In sexual addiction, some believe that individuals use the interpersonal dynamic of projective identification of sexuality for initiating and maintaining relationships. For individuals who use this relational style, the sexual projective identifications overshadow everything else; sex *is* the relationship rather than being a part of it (Cashdan, 1988). According to Cashdan, sexual addicts seem to use this style of relating to elicit others' perception of sexual excitement toward them. In this way, they do not necessarily objectify the other but view themselves as sexual objects.

A connection between sexual conditions with compulsive or addictive features and sexual infidelities recurring in ritualized patterns has been suggested by some researchers (Schneider, 1994; Schwartz & Masters, 1994). Certain key concepts in the individuals' behaviors, which are helpful in understanding addictive sexual disorders, include (1) loss of control over one or more sexual behaviors despite promises to oneself not to engage in them; (2) continuation of the behavior in the face of adverse consequences (loss of job or marriage, risk to safety, exposure to disease, etc.); (3) persistent pursuit of self-destructive behaviors; (4) spending a lot of time fantasizing about particular sexual activities; and (5) severe mood changes around sexual activities (Tays, Earle, Wells, Murray, & Garrett, 1999).

Some professionals disagree with the use of the term "sexual addiction" because no clear criteria have been established about what constitutes "normal" sexual involvement. Others argue that using the term "sexual addiction" takes advantage of people's fear of their own sexuality and pathologizes sexual behavior and impulses that are not unhealthy (Klein, 2003). Nevertheless, while avoiding the classification of sexual addiction, some professionals acknowledge that certain individuals do become engaged in patterns of excessive sexual activity that seem to reflect a lack of control.

For instance, sexologist Eli Coleman (2003) views these excessive sexual behaviors as symptomatic of sexual compulsion, a type of psychopathology (Coleman, 1995) rather than addiction. According to him, the individual involved in these behaviors suffers from feelings of inadequacy, shame, and loneliness. In order to relieve the psychological pain, the individual searches for a "fix"—an agent with pain-numbing qualities. After a brief respite from the pain, the individual then is again bombarded by the full force of the psychological pain he or she tried to escape.

The debate over excessive or uncontrolled sexuality and what to call it and how to treat it has found a new area of emphasis. Sex has become the most searched for topic among users of the internet, suggesting that a new variety of sexual compulsivity, *cybersex*, has evolved. Nationwide more than 2,000 treatment programs for compulsive or addictive sexual behaviors have emerged, most of them taking the 12-step program of Alcoholics Anonymous as their treatment model (National Council on Sexual Addiction and Compulsivity, 2002).

No matter what terminology or labels we use when describing or working with individuals who struggle with this type of difficulty, these activities—like most self-defeating behaviors—are expressions of the individuals' coping attempts to escape from the onslaught of the psychological pain they are experiencing.

Jenny: Pleasing Men To Feel Validated

Jenny grew up as the middle of three sisters in a middle-class family. All three girls adored their father and tried hard to please him. As psychological reasoning goes, the middle child in a family is the one who receives the least amount of attention from the parent, especially if all three siblings are of the same sex. Jenny, however, set out to disprove this hypothesis. Every bit of her behavior was designed and planned to please her father. Her hard work paid off; she became her father's favorite.

The lesson she retained for the rest of her life was to be validated by men. She married at an early age, gave birth to a daughter, and became successful in her nursing career. She enjoyed sexual activity with her husband and the attention she derived from it. Twelve years into the marriage, Jenny became bored. Sex with her husband now felt incestuous because he acted like a father. She had her first bout with depression.

Then the first of a series of extramarital affairs began. The antidepressant medication she was taking apparently, while reducing the degree of depression, increased her libido. She found an admiring young man. Life became exciting as Jenny embarked upon this affair. She observed him to learn what pleased him and supplied it. As the young man became dependent on her, Jenny felt powerful. She wondered if she could be as successful with other men. Soon another lover was added and another. For a while she managed to juggle all three, but eventually her husband found out. He threatened with divorce, Jenny asked for forgiveness, promised to end her affairs and remain faithful to her husband.

With the excitement of the affairs gone, depression returned. This time she had to be hospitalized because her psychiatrist declared her to be suicidal. Perhaps the medication had the same side effect as before: After release from the hospital Jenny's libido increased. Soon she found another lover. She made it her challenge to be the best lover in every man's life she ever got involved with. She craved the excitement of their desire for her. She needed their phone calls, their attention. This time her husband left when he found out; their daughter sided with him.

Jenny moved to another town, away from the reminders of her failed marriage. Living by herself, Jenny felt lonely, especially on her days off. As a nurse she worked several 12-hour days in a row, but then she might have 3 days off. She needed almost daily contacts from one of her lovers. Her sexual behavior was not only promiscuous, it became risky when she engaged in sex with men she hardly knew, just to ward off the loneliness. Hoping to regain her husband and daughter's sympathy, Jenny entered individual therapy. Of course, she was not a novice to therapy; over the years she had made her way through several treatment agencies. Some treatment professionals applied the label "sexual addiction" to her condition, while others considered her treatment regime within the category of personality disorders, still others treated her for a "chemical imbalance."

How did Jenny explain her sexual behaviors to herself? her therapist asked. Jenny described the process that started with feeling insecure, not important— perhaps even worthless. Those feelings naturally resulted in depression. To distract herself from the depression, she thought about ways she could make herself desirable to any man. As she fantasized about how to apply her skills, her mood improved and she felt a twinge of excitement. These preparatory fantasies included ritualistic elements. She felt powerful; "I know how to make a man feel important and special. As soon as he gets hooked on that feeling—and who wouldn't—he wants more and becomes dependent on me."

To Jenny, the men's level of dependence was a measure of her power and control. "In this whole process, what would you say are the most exciting moments for you?" the therapist asked. "Definitely the anticipation of how I get the man to the point of peak desire when he almost begs for me to let him have his way." Restating Jenny's words, "At that point you feel powerful because you could grant him his wish or could drop him on a bed of ice?" "Exactly," Jenny responded, "being in the position of granting him his moment of ecstasy or leaving him unfulfilled. I like your analogy of a 'bed of ice'; it increases the sense of power!"

"If the anticipation of your role in the sexual scenario excites you the most, how do you feel afterwards, when it's over for the evening?" Jenny thought for a moment before answering, "It's different at different times. Often I feel elated because I know I have given the man the absolute best sex he ever had. At other times I feel a bit let down because the guy—after having his climax—does not want to do much else and I am left hanging." "How do you cope with feeling 'left hanging'?" "That depends on whether I stay overnight with the man or not. If I stay, I may masturbate and hope for better sex in the morning. If I go home, I take a shower and go to bed. I usually don't masturbate then because I feel too bad about the experience. I may have a glass of wine to calm me down for sleep."

"Now that you and your husband have separated, are you considering any of the men you have been with as a permanent partner?" Jenny sounded surprised, "Do you mean marrying one of them?" "Yes, that would be a possibility, wouldn't it?" Jenny seemed to explore the prospect, "Well, there are one or two that I would consider interesting for their intellectual power, but neither one would make it easy to live with. They are set in their ways and I would not want to accommodate to that. Some of the others I could not imagine myself spending my whole day with; we have too little in common for that."

The therapist continued to explore the reality of Jenny's involvement. "You seem to think that the men who are intellectually stimulating would not make changes in their lifestyles to accommodate you and those who you find less interesting would not qualify for an expanded relationship—what exactly is in it for you, pleasing these different men?" "That's a question I have asked myself and I don't have a good answer," Jenny replied, "When I think about an upcoming sexual encounter I get excited about the role I am going to play and, of course, I anticipate an outcome to my liking."

"Which would be ...?" Jenny's answer sounded like she was considering a dream, "The man—although he could have any other woman—is so infatuated with me that he cannot think of anything but pleasing me and being with me every moment of his life. Nothing else would matter in his life." "Has this happened?" the therapist inquired gently. "No, and I am afraid it never will, but I have to keep trying." "Why?" "My life would be meaningless without it."

The question at the end of this therapy session remains: Is Jenny's sexual desire really "sexual" or is it part of an obsessive-compulsive disorder, or does it constitute an addiction? In addition, some of her responses seem to indicate a histrionic quality to her personality. On the other hand, the excitement of being powerful and in control that she interprets as a sexual high—even though she uses her control skills mainly to assure that the men have the greatest experiences of their life—is this merely the expression of her need to be affirmed as a worthwhile human being or is it a drive for control despite competition with other women? Jenny could not make that distinction yet.

Cashdan's (1988) notion of sexual projective identification by using the promissory gift of sexual excitement to initiate relationships could also be applicable to explain Jenny's interpersonal dynamics and behaviors as she is working hard to give the man the "absolute best sex he ever had."

Some professionals might want to consider Jenny's case in terms of the power and control aspects, which seem to afford her a high level of excitement. And certainly, that is a valid point. As can be seen in Chapter 6, power seems to hold an almost sexual interest for some women, either by holding the power themselves or "borrowing" the power—by being close to the source of it. Some of the women's stories could be explored under various characteristic categories simultaneously. Usually, people do not fit neatly into just one category; they are too complicated for that.

PART II
The Women in Context

4
Searching for Sexual Identity

In an earlier part of the book (Chapter 1), during the discussion of how cultural factors shape sexual desire, the story of the young southern woman Melanie who discovered sexual desire after years of marriage was used for illustration. Through cognitive-behavioral therapy Melanie had been able to explore and challenge the logic of her underlying beliefs about women of her background not being encouraged to enjoy sexual activities. When she allowed herself to relax during sexual activities and focus on her physical sensations, she was surprised to feel desire and arousal for the first time in her life. She could hardly believe what she and Gregory had missed out on for so long—only because she did not know better. Melanie made it her goal to educate her friends and relatives about her discovery. Gregory paid a visit to the sex therapist. With a big smile on his face and a beautiful bouquet of flowers in his arms, he expressed his happiness and gratitude. Life had become exciting again as he felt warm and secure in Melanie's love for him.

Melanie's story demonstrates the difficulty women encounter in trying to define for themselves the nature of their sexual being. For many women it is difficult enough to define themselves in terms of womanhood. Should they become sophisticated career women, should they be satisfied with being their mate's helper, should they opt for being the strong earth mother who gives birth to and raises healthy and well-adjusted children—or should they be all of that? When they grow into the type of womanhood chosen for themselves—or just as often by others—what type of sexual being will fit their image of themselves as the "total woman?"

Adolescence and the Formation of Sexual Identity

Adolescence is the time to develop a sense of identity in preparation for the task of establishing intimacy with another. Psychoanalyst Erik Erikson (1950), who called this time in a young person's life the "identity versus role confusion" stage, proposed that real intimacy with another person was possible only once a sense of identity has been developed. Only when the young girl feels secure in her identity can she truly share herself with another person.

Most adolescents by age 12 or 13 have a basic notion of what it means to be "in love." Interestingly, by the end of adolescence, the average boy believes having been in love more often than the average girl even though the progression toward romantic relationships occurs faster for girls (Montgomery & Sorel, 1997). Furthermore, girls—in contrast to boys—seem to regard romantic relationships as a context for self-disclosure (Feiring, 1999). This gender difference does not seem to change significantly during the rest of the lifespan development.

Much of the current work on the formation of adolescent identity grew out of James Marcia's description of *identity statuses*, influenced by Erikson's general conceptions of the adolescent identity process. Marcia (1966, 1980) proposed that adolescent identity formation consists of two parts: a crisis and a commitment. The crisis part is a period of decision-making—usually during an upheaval— when values are reexamined. As a result of the reevaluation, the young person makes a commitment to a specific value, goal, role, or ideology.

In Marcia's conceptualization, four different identity statuses are possible: the *identity achievement*, which is the status when after the crisis resolution the individual has committed to ideological, occupational, or other goals. During the *moratorium*, the individual is in an upheaval but has not made a commitment. A person who has accepted and committed to parental or culturally defined norms without having gone through a crisis is in the *foreclosure* status. Those who are not in a crisis and who have not yet made a commitment are the ones that experience *identity diffusion*.

Today, for many girls the quest for sexual identity may come well before the search for their personal female identity. Adolescents are concerned with the way their peers evaluate them. To be accepted into the right group of popular girls, it is not only important to wear the right clothes, to choose the right hairstyle, but also to have a boyfriend. Of course, boyfriends are also rated according to their popularity and the girls' standing in their group is related to their boyfriends' level of popularity.

Cultural influences in general encourage girls and young women to spend more time, money, and effort on looking and *appearing* sexy than on *being* sexy. Appearing sexy is for the benefit of another—the boyfriend or man they want to attract. Appearing sexy operates out of an other-focused mindset. On the other hand, being sexy is for oneself, to enjoy one's own sexual feelings and fulfillment; it is part of a self-oriented mindset.

Some research indicated that there is a difference in the way males and females experience the adolescent/early adulthood crisis (Lytle, Bakken, & Romig, 1997; Moretti & Wiebe, 1999). Girls seem to follow Erikson's and Marcia's hypotheses about adolescent identity formation better than boys. At a younger age than boys, girls are thought to consolidate their identities by integrating their internal beliefs about themselves with information obtained from others in their social relationships. Boys, on the other hand, are thought to focus more on internal sources and beliefs than on social sources of information and thus take a longer time for their identity achievement.

One could argue, however, that instead of reaching identity achievement earlier, girls are actually delaying the process by following—rather than truly integrating—the information gained through social relationships. Their true identity formation might occur at a much later time when they are awakening to the reality of some of the consequences from earlier commitments made under the influence of social sources.

Self-Esteem and Peer Pressure

A significant factor in the developmental process is the individual's self-esteem because it influences not only aspired levels of achievement but also selection of friends and romantic-sexual attachments. Researchers have looked at the stability of adolescents' self-esteem ratings and have divided them into four categories (Diehl, Vicary, & Deike, 1997; Zimmerman, Copeland, Shope, & Dielman, 1997). They found that throughout adolescence about half of the adolescents in their studies displayed consistently high self-esteem. Those in the second group showed steady increases in self-esteem, while the self-esteem ratings in the third group remained consistently low. Individuals in the fourth group appeared to possess moderate to high self-esteem at the beginning of the period but there was a steady decline as adolescence progressed.

These findings raised concerns as it was revealed that females outnumbered males in the third and fourth categories (Zimmerman et al., 1997). Given that adolescents with high self-esteem are not only more focused on achievement, but they are also better able to resist peer pressure, the concern is well-founded.

Acceptance and Standing Within Their Own Circles

As the girl's connection to being accepted is often the type of boys that are attracted to her, the mechanism by which to maintain the link to the boyfriend is by way of sex. And although for the past several years the overall percentage of high-school students having sexual intercourse declined somewhat for all grades, non-coital sexual expression has become a common sexual behavior among adolescents. In particular, oral-genital stimulation among teenagers has increased dramatically and is now two to three times more frequent than was reported in the Kinsey studies (Woody, Russel, D'Souza, & Woody, 2000). Some young people prefer this type of sexual activity because technically they are still able to remain virgins.

Does Oral-Genital Stimulation Count as Sex?

Some young people do not even regard oral-genital stimulation as sex, an informal survey of young college students revealed. In fact, for another group of students, a new type of entertainment among high-school students seems to be an event called "Rainbow Parties." Female high-school students wearing different-colored lipstick perform fellatio on the boys at the party. As the saliva from the girls' mouths smoothes the edges of the lipstick colors of the girls who performed fellatio on the same boy before them, the exterior of the boy's penis is said to resemble a rainbow.

One can find discussions and opinions about this practice on the internet, dating back to 2003 when a guest on the Oprah show talked about it. More recently a novel for teenagers was published with the title *Rainbow Party*. Many of the discussants doubt the actual existence of these rainbow parties, calling them a new urban legend rather than reality. But even so, although it might have started out as a fake, it is only a small step to making it a reality; and according to some concerned mothers, the practice has already caught on in some areas of the country.

It is difficult to say what and how these practices contribute to the formation of a girl's sexual identity. The tremendous pressure many girls encounter when they are trying to attract and keep a boyfriend leaves them little energy or opportunity to explore what they might want out of a sexual relationship.

Menstrual Shame and Sexual Attitudes

Although the event of menarche brings about excitement in many young girls because it signals a step into womanhood, for others this natural process evokes shame. There is still a cultural taboo among us that menstruation is something not to be discussed openly, to be kept hidden as if it were a dirty and disgusting event. This shame about menstruation often includes discomfort about the vagina and surrounding areas, which many women regard as unpleasant and ugly (Braun & Wilkinson, 2001). Thus, shame about menstruation extends to shame about one's body in general for many girls and young women.

In many young women's minds, menarche is also connected to the emerging sexual potential developing in the woman, and the attitudes about menstruation the young girl holds might impact her developing sexual attitudes and the sexual decisions she makes. Several researchers have looked at specific links between menstrual attitudes and both sexual attitudes and sexual behavior. For instance, in one study undergraduate women who acknowledged feeling more comfortable with menstruation also reported more comfort with their sexuality and an increased likelihood of engaging in sexual intercourse while menstruating (Rempel & Baumgartner, 2003).

Another study with undergraduate women revealed that those women who reported shame about menstruation also reported less sexual activity. However, when they did engage in sexual activity, they admitted to participating in more sexual risk-taking (Schooler, 2001). Reinholtz and Muehlenhard (1995) found that undergraduate women who perceived their genitals to be dirty, smelly, and shameful seemed to engage less in sexual activities and reported less enjoyment of sexual activity.

It would not be surprising to find a connection between menstrual and genital shame on the one hand and reduced sexual activity and enjoyment on the other. If one is ashamed of a part of one's body, then it would stand to reason that one would hesitate to display it to the participant/observer in sexual intercourse; and the shame would interfere with any kind of enjoyment that could be derived from the activity.

In order to investigate the impact of menstrual shame and global body shame on sexual decision-making, Schooler, Ward, Merriwether, and Caruthers (2005) reasoned that shame about menstruation has an effect on a global sense of body shame and thus indirectly influences sexual attitudes and behavior. The investigators focused on shame rather than on body dissatisfaction because shame involves not only negative evaluations of one's body but also an emotional component, the desire to hide one's body. The desire to hide may not always be included in body dissatisfaction. Additionally, body shame includes more than body size and shape—aspects involved in body dissatisfaction—but also contains factors such as smells and body hair.

The sample population for the investigators' study consisted of 199 female students from an undergraduate psychology class, ranging in age from 17 years to 23 years. Measures were obtained through self-rating instruments completed by the participants. For the assessment of menstrual attitudes, three subscales from the post-menarcheal version of the Adolescent Menstrual Attitude Questionnaire (Morse, Kieren, & Bottorff, 1993) tapping *negative feelings, positive feelings* and including an *openness* subscale were used.

To assess the degree of body shame, the investigators used the Body Comfort/Body Modesty Measure (BCBM) (Merriwether & Ward, 2002), a scale containing 29 items focusing on one's comfort with the appearance and function of one's body. Another measure, the Body Image Self-Consciousness Scale (BISC) (Wiederman, 2000), was used to assess body shame in intimate situations. Sexual assertiveness was selected as the primary sexual outcome.

Among their findings the investigators reported that—as had been expected—women who acknowledged more negative attitudes related to menstruation reported significantly less sexual assertiveness. Those women who endorsed openness about menstruation also acknowledged significantly more sexual assertiveness as well as more sexual experience. No direct relationship was found between positive feelings about menstruation and the sexual outcome variables.

Analyzing the data regarding menstrual attitudes and body shame, again it was found that women with negative attitudes about menstruation also reported feeling more self-conscious about their body image, whereas women with open attitudes toward menstruation experienced less self-consciousness about their body image.

Partial correlations between the two body shame measures and the four sexual outcomes (sexual assertiveness, sexual experience, sexual risk, and condom self-efficacy) indicated that greater body comfort predicted higher levels of sexual assertiveness, higher levels of sexual experience, lower levels of sexual risk-taking behaviors, and greater condom use self-efficacy. On the other hand, greater self-consciousness about body image was linked to lower levels of sexual assertiveness and sexual experience as well as lower condom use self-efficacy.

In their discussion of the findings the authors acknowledged that their expectations regarding the connections between menstrual attitudes, body shame, and various aspects of sexual behaviors had been confirmed, but they cautioned that cause-and-effect conclusions should not be automatically assumed because other factors may be involved that need further exploration. For instance, while women's body attitudes may interfere with sexual assertiveness and sexual behavior, it is also possible that their sexual experiences—how their partners appear to evaluate their bodies during sexual activity—shape the women's attitudes about and comfort with their bodies.

Women's Fantasies About the Man in Their Future Instead of Their Own Sexual Identity

In general, it is probably safe to say that women spend more time thinking and fantasizing about the man they expect to love and be loved by than about their own sexual moves and activities once the man has arrived on the scene. Romanticizing these aspects of life might give the fantasy a wonderful overall glow, but it does not lead to specifying particular aspects that take on relevance in actual life.

Irene: Permanent Scars

Irene, a girl with a beautiful face and beautiful voice, was envied by many of her friends. She was an attentive listener and her smile made everybody around her feel good. Everybody agreed: Irene had a friendly, caring, and pleasing personality. What people did not know was that she had a physical disfigurement that was deeply disturbing to her. She could hide it under clothing but she knew that if she ever entered a physically intimate relationship, to a lover or husband, her deformity would be obvious immediately. Her fears related to the eventual discovery of her defect were not conducive to great explorations of her sexual identity although she occasionally indulged in fantasies of a romantic nature, like many of her friends did.

In accordance with Schooler et al.'s (2005) findings that greater self-consciousness or shame about body image correlates with lower levels of sexual assertiveness and sexual experience, Irene married the first young man who asked her. Her disclosure had been somewhat less traumatic than she had feared in her worst imagination, but she never forgot it. Although she gave birth to four children in rather short succession, she did not enjoy sex. She could never relax enough to soak up some of the good sensations that come from two bodies touching, and she never experienced an orgasm. Irene's husband became a successful attorney and with the enhanced financial resources his work brought and improved medical technology, Irene could afford corrective surgery. Although the surgery was a success, Irene's concept of herself did not improve. The scar resulting from the surgery was still a visible reminder of her imperfection.

Media's Role in Girls' Transformation Into Women

Information on how to transform themselves from girls into young women according to cultural standards of the time can be found in the media and especially in teen magazines (McRobbie, 1991). The main focus of teen magazines seems to be directed toward fashion, entertainment, and beauty hints; products that promise to improve one's attractiveness and love life; and in the past two decades toward topics dealing with sexuality. Adolescence is the time when young people learn what is appropriate sexually as they are being exposed to many cultural-level scripts and expectations. Adolescence is also a time when young people are most impressionable and what has been presented to them by the media may affect their values, beliefs, attitudes, and behaviors throughout their lifetimes. Teen magazines, by virtue of their popularity, are great vehicles to disseminate cultural-level scripts on sexuality as well as many other issues of the time.

Seventeen

As one of the oldest and most widely read of the teen magazines, *Seventeen* was chosen by researcher Laura Carpenter (1998) to analyze changes in the magazine's depiction of sexuality over a 20-year period ending in 1994. Carpenter pointed out that the range of sexual scripts available in *Seventeen* expanded to recognize and include issues such as female sexual desire, ambivalence about sexuality, masturbation, oral sex, homosexuality, and recreational sex. But as Carpenter emphasized, in general, the editors of the magazine resolved controversial issues in ways that reinforced culturally dominant gender and sexual norms. For instance, by discussing recreational sex scenarios while at the same time presenting traditional sexual scenarios and urging young women to abstain from sexual intercourse, the editors can claim that several sides of an issue have been explored. But by emphasizing the traditional script, they may leave the reader in a state of ambiguity or confusion.

Exploration and analysis of the magazine issues left the investigator with the impression that the editors rarely selected items from the current events and social problems that are normally covered in news magazines. Rather, the content of issues appeared to be determined by seasonal merchandizing requirements. Not surprisingly, advertisers' interests seemed to exert the greatest control over the content of teen magazines (McCracken, 1993).

Among the changes occurring in *Seventeen* from 1974 to 1994, the investigator found that the magazine's editors were depicting young women as proactive individuals who experience sexual desires (in contrast to previous portrayals as sexual objects and victims). Other changes included recognition of young women's ambivalence about sexuality as well as more positive editorial positions toward masturbation, homosexuality, and the acknowledgement of fellatio—although cunnilingus was not mentioned. Even while presenting these topics, editors maintained their favorable stance with regard to established sexual scripts.

Another change that could be observed was that by 1994 scenarios with acknowledgement of sexual desires and the fulfillment of those desires had become more prominent. Regarding sex within a recreational context, statements such as, "a love relationship is not absolutely necessary for sexual activities but all sexual activities are enjoyed more within a loving, trusting, committed relationship," convey a double-sided message.

The aspect of individual morality, which stresses the rights of young women to make choices about sexual behavior based on their own beliefs, was a consistent characteristic of the magazine's content over the time period explored by the investigator. By encouraging women to make choices congruent with their beliefs, the individual morality scripts depicted women as determining agents of their behaviors. However, suggestions of avoiding sexual activity rather than seeking it followed with warnings that the dangers of sex outweigh the potential pleasures seems to discourage women's role as active participant. Thus, young women may experience desire, but the fulfillment of these desires is wrought with danger unless acting on the desire is postponed to the distant future.

The notion that desire and pleasure are problematic for women seems reminiscent of Vance's (1989) writings. For women, the expression of sexual desire comes with two consequences: One is the danger of rape, or of pregnancy, and of harassment because men will interpret women's expression of desire as an invitation for sexual activity. In addition, by expressing desire women are signaling that they are giving up their traditional responsibility as "gate-keepers" of sexuality and with that their control of sex. They are violating the traditional feminine role.

Considering the dangers of rape, pregnancy, and harassment as consequences of women expressing their sexual desire would logically lead to a repression of sexual desire in most women. Thus, the implied threat of "victim-blaming" exerts a dampening influence on women's sexuality.

Pornography

As if this were not enough, most erotica and pornographic materials that are supposed to be sexually arousing are targeted toward men, because men are the best customers for these items. It is hardly by accident that these materials tend to present pictures of women that are the ultimate in physical beauty and at the same time passive objects of men's pleasure. The body is emphasized over the person. Women are simultaneously idealized in terms of physical appearance and belittled by being objectified (Lips, 2005).

The requirements of physical beauty may leave women with a significant dent in their self-esteem and the portrayed passivity is not congruent with an expression of felt sexual desire. In addition, these sexually oriented materials seem to focus increasingly on brutalization and degradation of women, which serves to reinforce the myths of men's sexual dominance and women's sexual passivity and powerlessness.

People may not always agree on what aspects of pornographic presentations render the scenes as acts of degradation. Most popular videos seem to include sexually explicit behavior, casual sex, behaviors of dominance (such as ignoring the wishes of a sexual partner), submission, objectification (treating one partner as object or plaything), as well as a form of penis/semen worship (sexual activity focusing on the penis and ejaculation).

In a study exploring the possible objectification of women in pornographic videos in Australia (McKee, 2005), the majority of videos used were American imports. Raters were trained to observe the existence of several variables contained in the videos. It was found that of the 642 scenes that contained sexual activities, 198 showed sex being initiated by women and 110 being initiated by men. In 47 of the scenes sex had been initiated by all participants, and the majority (287) of the scenes opened after sex had already been initiated. In 51 cases, all characters seemed to experience orgasm, whereas in 436 cases only the male characters had orgasms, compared with 25 cases where only women appeared to experience orgasm, mostly through penile/vaginal penetration.

The most popular sex act presented in the scenes was that of penile/vaginal penetration. In the scenes depicting oral sex, it was more common for women to perform oral sex on the male characters. The investigator mentioned that the appearance of women initiating sex more often in the pornographic videos might provide an unrealistic vision of women's sexuality. Additionally, the fact that women were depicted far more often than men performing oral sex could represent an overvaluing of male over female sexual pleasure in these videos, according to the investigator.

The majority of the male characters' orgasms were apparently achieved through masturbation and 32 of the orgasms (22.5%) experienced by the female characters also were achieved through masturbation. The interpretation that this focus on female orgasm through masturbation represented a concern for female sexual pleasure in these videos could also be viewed as just another way to arouse male observers, since it is known that female masturbation and female–female sexual activities contain aspects of arousal for male viewers. Perhaps more realistic opinions could be obtained from those individuals who actually view these videos for their own purposes than from the researcher-trained coders. After all, the consumer is the ultimate judge of what appeals to him or her and why.

A surprising finding of the study was the discovery that the majority of videos containing sexually violent scenes apparently had been targeted specifically at the female audience. However, it was not clear from the study whether the videotapes targeted for the female audience were indeed purchased or rented mainly by female consumers or male consumers.

Lenore: Shocked by Pornography

As the younger of two sisters, Lenore was considered by her family to be a free spirit both in thought and action. While in college she experimented with her own sexuality and felt independent and equal to the young men she dated. She was as ambitious as they were and she was outspoken about her goals and wishes. After graduation from college she embarked upon a career in the medical field. At a social gathering she spotted the man who she felt was to be her future husband. Her feelings were so strong and convincing that she approached him with the words, "You should marry me." The object of her directive, Howard, handled his surprise well and responded, "In that case, you should join me for dinner."

This was the beginning of a brief, intense, and passionate dating relationship. After about 8 weeks they got married. Although Lenore learned that Howard had been married before, she did not inquire about the reasons for the divorce of Howard's first marriage. She was convinced that their meeting was an act of destiny; she did not need additional information. It was almost 2 years after the date of their first meeting that Lenore gave birth to twin daughters. Lenore had everything she wanted: a wonderful husband, two lovely little girls, and a successful career.

Three years later Lenore confided in a friend that Howard was watching pornography on the computer in his study. Her friend asked if Lenore knew what kind of pornography he was watching, but Lenore did not seem interested or bothered by it. To her friend's expressed concern about the situation Lenore responded with, "I don't mind if he gets all fired up sexually as long as he uses his excitement with me. Our sex life seems to benefit from this."

One evening after the children were asleep Lenore entered Howard's study. She observed him, as his eyes seemed glued to the screen while his hand was fondling his penis. The images on the screen shocked her into an emotional vacuum. She quietly left the room and Howard never noticed her presence. Later that night Howard initiated sex. Lenore seemed numb and unable to respond in her usual active manner. It was one of the few times in their relationship that she did not achieve an orgasm. It also seemed to her that Howard was more rough than usual in his lovemaking. She thought that this had occurred before but she had always explained it as an expression of his passionate love for her.

At the occasion of their next lovemaking, Lenore could not prevent some of the images she had seen on the computer screen that evening from invading her mind. No matter how hard she tried to concentrate on Howard's touch and his arousal, the images kept popping up in her mind. Howard noticed the difference in her, but she was able to make up an excuse about not feeling well. She decided that it might help in the future if she had a little more wine than usual at dinner to keep those images away. As the images persisted Lenore's alcohol intake increased until she was close to the point of passing out. She had used the alcohol to keep her from remembering the pornographic scenes, but it also reduced her sensuousness and sex became devoid of emotions or physical sensations.

The realization that she was on her way to becoming an alcoholic scared Lenore into talking to Howard. He seemed sorry that she had been so uncomfortable about his watching pornography and suggested that she might get over the discomfort by watching it with him. Lenore refused that invitation and requested his promise that he would not indulge in it again. His promise sounded a bit weak but Lenore accepted it.

Weeks went by during which Lenore tried to engage in romantic fantasies to get her sexual interest started again. However, when her fantasies turned to some of their past sexual interactions, the pornographic images sneaked in and turned desire into disgust. Her fantasies turned into negative relational representations, antifantasies, as described by Kaplan (see Chapter 3). Without the numbing effect of the alcohol, her mind was not able to relax as it had in the safety of their early lovemaking. The repugnant imaginings eliminated any feelings of sexual desire within the context of sexual activities with her husband. She wondered what Howard was thinking of her when they engaged in sexual activities after he had been watching pornography. Was she the same as the degraded and objectified female bodies on the screen, meant to endure passively the defiling and invasion of her body?

Then came an evening when Howard seemed to spend a long time in his study. Lenore was scared of her own suspicion, but she walked into his room. This time Howard heard her. He pulled her close and forced her to watch the pornography with him for a while. Then he pulled her head down and forced her to perform oral sex on him while he continued to watch the screen. When he let go of her, Lenore was nauseated and ran into the bathroom where she spent several hours. Finally she went to sleep in her daughters' room.

The next morning, before getting ready for work, she asked Howard to leave the house but she packed a few things for herself and her daughters in case Howard would ignore her request. At work she contacted an attorney; Howard had agreed to move out. During the process of divorce Lenore learned that Howard's addiction to pornography had been the reason for the divorce from his first wife. Although Lenore would have liked to share her life with another man, she was unable to overcome the disgust and repulsion she experienced when thinking about sex. She was close to developing a sexual aversion disorder, and she was not sure that she could ever trust another man.

Finally she entered therapy to help her resolve her panic about sex. She knew she had to be able to provide a healthy sexual attitude for her daughters. Lenore recognized that the strong conviction of her own feelings about her fateful meeting with Howard had kept her from obtaining important information about the person she was to share her life with. She paid a high price for her refusal to know more about the man of her dreams. As her dream turned into a nightmare, she had come close to self-destruction with the increased use of alcohol as a coping mechanism to block out the revolting images. And she had lost the healthy vital sexual desire she once possessed.

Influence of Sex Education Curricula

Messages in the popular media as well as sex education curricula most likely will be perceived as irrelevant if they contradict young women's actual experiences. Sex education scripts that do not acknowledge female desire foster confusion in young women instead of preparing them for making sexual decisions (Tolman, 1994). It is unlikely that young women will benefit from sex education curricula that do not make efforts to disentangle romance and sexuality (Thompson, 1995).

In 1996, the U.S. Congress allocated $250 million to fund school-based "abstinence only" programs over the next 5 years. In order to be eligible for a part of this federal grant, state abstinence-only programs, among other mandated topics, had to emphasize the social, psychological, and health benefits which would be gained by abstaining from sexual activity. The expected standard for all school-age children was total sexual abstinence outside of marriage, and the only absolutely sure way to prevent out-of-wedlock pregnancy and health problems related to sexual activity was to remain sexually abstinent (Koch, 1998).

Some of the young people who adhere to the ideal of chastity until marriage refuse to think about sexuality, perhaps fearing that thinking and talking about sex might result in too much temptation to break the vows of abstinence. Colleges and universities today provide classes in marriage and family as well as in human sexuality as part of the regular course work. Instructors of these classes are sometimes faced with young students who disagree with discussing sexual aspects of marriage, insisting that when the time comes to get married their love and their faith will make everything just right.

On the other hand, refusing to obtain information about sexual matters is not a successful approach to establishing one's sexual identity. Sex therapists have worked with clients who were virgins on their wedding night and as a result not everything was going well. For some, the anxiety about what to do left them paralyzed with tension or too anxious to have or maintain an erection.

Fear of pain when a penis is about to be inserted into the woman's vagina for the first time might lead to spasms that make penetration impossible, and the woman may suffer from vaginismus, a condition of strong involuntary contractions of the muscles in the outer third of the vagina, for some time. An estimated 2% of women suffer from vaginismus. Not all women who experience vaginismus are sexually unresponsive; some of them enjoy sex play and are orgasmic with manual and oral stimulation. However, there are also accounts of couples not having consummated their marriage 5 to 20 years or more after their wedding.

Cathy: Virgin Bride

Cathy married at the age of 19 while she was still in training as X-ray technician. She was a virgin and had had practically no sex education. Ted, her young husband, had consulted some of his male friends, and, although he was several years older than Cathy, his sexual knowledge was limited. They succeeded in having sexual intercourse on their wedding night but it was not a pleasant experience. Due to the excitement and, no doubt some anxiety, Ted climaxed almost immediately after penetration. Besides the slight burning pain that accompanied the breaking of her hymen, Cathy felt nothing.

Future attempts at sex did not improve significantly. Cathy was disappointed but the birth of her daughters more than made up for it—she thought. She did not complain. Ted's sex drive was strong, but his techniques did not improve, possibly because there were no complaints from Cathy, who dreaded sex and tried to put it off as long as she could. Strong resentment built up between the two of them and they finally divorced.

Through her work in the medical field, Cathy became friends with a few of the nurses she met and confided in them that she felt inadequate to help her daughters with sexual issues when they would ask questions about it. The nurses recommended a few books for her to read. Cathy realized that she had been missing out on some pleasurable experiences; she learned to masturbate and found herself engaged in erotic fantasies. However, she was frightened by her own fantasies and did not disclose them to anybody. She was convinced that her fantasies were sinful and perverted.

After a few years Cathy married again and sex between her and her new husband was better than it had been with Ted, but she did not allow herself to enjoy her husband's caresses. If his actions resembled anything in her fantasies, her body became rigid and unresponsive. Her sexual desire, which had been awakened to a degree by the newness of the relationship and the influence of her fantasies, was stifled again because she tried to suppress her feelings. She could not possibly share the content of her fantasies with her husband; he would be appalled, she feared.

Cathy had the opportunity to attend a professional conference in another part of the country. It was exciting to travel by herself and stay in a big hotel. On the last evening of the conference she entered the hotel's bar and looked around. She was about to leave when one of the men sitting at the bar got up and invited her to join him for a drink. Cathy accepted the invitation and stayed for several drinks. After that she accompanied the man to his room. The alcohol loosened her inhibitions and she participated actively in their sex play and even allowed herself to play out some of her fantasies. She had never been so aroused in her life. They fell asleep exhaustedly. At about four o'clock in the morning Cathy woke up, naked, next to a stranger. She quickly got dressed, went to her room, packed her belongings, and went straight to the airport. Her flight home was not due to leave until the early afternoon but she felt safer at the airport than in the hotel where she might run into the man from the night before.

While waiting at the airport, Cathy was on an emotional roller-coaster—shock, fear, disgust, guilt, along with some strange sensuous feeling bombarded her. How could she have agreed to have sex with a total stranger—even worse—how could she have enjoyed it? What would her husband think if he found out? What if she became pregnant? Her husband had undergone a vasectomy before they met and therefore there had not been any need for birth control considerations. What if she had picked up a sexually transmitted disease? Cathy had many hours to worry about those questions.

Once in her familiar surroundings, she tried to forget the dangerous adventure. There had been no catastrophic consequences. Unfortunately, the experience had not brought about an increased sexual desire when she was with her husband. If she had let go of her inhibitions with him, how could she face him afterward? In her opinion, this was not the kind of woman he married.

A little more than a year later another conference brought with it another opportunity. Cathy told herself that she would not repeat her previous experience. But as soon as she had settled in her seat in the airplane, she started thinking about the sexual encounter and her own fantasies until she actually became aroused and finally went to the restroom to masturbate. She knew she was going to repeat last year's experience and she did.

This time she confessed to her husband upon her return home. After the initial shock had worn off and the angry outbursts had made room for some calmer contemplation, he suggested they both participate in marital and sex therapy. Cathy's husband accepted part of the responsibility for Cathy's sexual inhibition while with him. He had been unaware of her thoughts and desires in her fantasies. It was his wish to help channel Cathy's hidden desires into their lovemaking.

During therapy sessions, the underlying beliefs that triggered her inhibitions were explored and brought into Cathy's awareness. As an adjunct to therapy, videos proved an effective tool for the couple's work. Some of the videos Cathy would watch by herself before agreeing to see them with her husband; others he would bring home and suggest they watch together. Cathy's husband made sure to communicate his excitement over her expressions of arousal and interest in exploring various positions and roles in their sex play. He encouraged her to create scenes from her fantasies that they could reenact together.

From Cathy's story, we observe that sexual desire can be present in some situations and not in others, as it may be experienced with some partners but not with others—all within the same woman. Although situational factors provide their own impact and partner characteristics and behavior influence a woman's sexual feelings and wishes, her own cognitive framework, her own attitudes and beliefs, are often the most significant determinants of her sexual experiences. The role she adopts for herself provides the framework for her life's path.

Transformation From Woman to Wife

When dating with the intent to marry, women understand that sex will be part of the relationship, at least insofar as it is a requirement for parenthood. This understanding does not lead to discussions beyond perhaps how many children to include in the family. With the achievement of the desired number of children, sex loses its importance in many women's minds. Women often do not think about marriage in terms beyond romance and motherhood. As one young woman said, "When you think of getting married you know that you will have sex because you want to have children. While you are focusing on getting pregnant, you don't even realize whether you enjoy sex or not; it's part of life. After having the children that you wanted, there is no need to have sex. It's something I never thought about in detail."

In her book *Marriage Shock,* Dalma Heyn (1997) gave a description of the process of transformation that many women undergo when they become wives. Girls and women change themselves into what they have come to believe wives should be like. In the transformation what initially was exciting and enjoyable to themselves and their husbands might have gotten lost. They don't allow themselves the luxury of reaching for what they want. "Good wives" are not supposed to be selfish and asking for what you desire would seem a selfish thing to do.

Even women whose behavior demonstrates a certain degree of selfishness are often hard put to answer questions like "What do you want?" or "What would please you?" because they refuse to verbalize any self-pleasing thoughts to others and often even to themselves. In the process of following the expected behavioral rules for the "good wife" women become estranged from themselves.

In the sexual area of life women, more often than not, follow the lead of the men they are with. Men are still the initiators, and women let them determine the pace and sequence in the process of sexual intercourse. Men, of course, will proceed in a manner that they are accustomed to and feel comfortable with. Often, as part of the transition to wife, a previously significant element of the couple's interaction gets lost.

Seduction, which previously was used to ignite the spark of sexual interest and desire, unfortunately, gradually disappears from many long-term monogamous relationships, as Lonnie Barbach (1999) pointed out in her introduction to the book *Seduction: Tales of Erotic Persuasion*. Barbach regards this as a tragic loss because the sexual liveliness and passion of the previous interactions will be replaced by occupation with the mundane, which diminishes the quality of the relationship.

Seduction is a game with two interacting partners, both of whom are willing to continue playing to various levels. As either partner is in a position to determine the level of escalation at any given moment, women can take this as opportunity to teach their partners how and when to play the game of seduction. Unfortunately, this opportunity is often left unused when women choose to be less active in the dance of seduction.

The Goal of Orgasm

In some relationships, the sexual interaction is gender-based in an "orgasm versus intimacy" framework. In general, the climax is the ultimate goal of sexual activity for men, but this is not necessarily the case for women. With that arrangement, women agree to participate sexually in men's sexual styles instead of their own and chances are slim that women get what they want.

Men and women's sexuality and attitudes about sex are not the same. In fact, there is a difference expressed in their attitudes about masturbation. When men complain in the therapist's office about the low frequency of sex in the marriage, the therapist may inquire about masturbation. More often than not, the man will respond that he should not need to do that since he is in a permanent relationship. Women, on the other hand, unless their sexual interest is nonexistent, will more readily report that they masturbate—even while they are in a committed relationship.

Masturbation is a safe way for women to learn about orgasm. In the privacy of their bedroom or bathroom they learn how to achieve it and how it feels when they experience it. Sometimes they learn so well that they can give convincing performances with their partners. Eileen had "faked" orgasms all through her marriage. She loved her husband but did not like his style of lovemaking and the behavioral demands he placed on her. In order to reduce the time spent in activities she did not care for, she utilized her "orgasm performance." The problem arose when after 14 years of "faking" she was tired of it. In fact, her performance backfired: the high quality of her orgasms encouraged her husband to increase his demands for the activities she did not want to perform. He felt justified to request the fulfillment of his preferences because he had given her so much pleasure over the years. What was Eileen to do? She could not possibly let her husband know that she had been dishonest.

It is generally believed that women associate sex with love but for men that association is often not necessary. Are women finding the longed-for expression of love in men's sexual behavior if they let men go ahead according to their own plans? That is not very likely because men don't know in detail what women are looking for as expressions of love—beyond the statement "I love you." And why should they? It is women's responsibility to make their wishes known and understood.

The more women allow themselves to participate in interactions that are not pleasing to them—even if they do it because they want to please their partners—the more they will get of what they don't want. It is also not quite fair to a man to let him proceed blindly according to his notion of sexual enjoyment and then resent him for not reading the woman's mind and fulfilling her unexpressed wishes and expectations. Thus, by adopting the idealized picture of the "good wife" who is able to care for everybody's needs and happiness—except her own—at the end of the day the woman falls into bed exhausted from conducting her multitask life without energy left for any playful sexual encounters.

The Trap of "Multitasking"

"Multitasking" is a popular word for today's wives and mothers and everybody supports them in their striving for multitask achievements. Nancy, a young mother of three children, wondered why she was not as efficient as the other young women in her neighborhood. They seemed to be able to deal with all kinds of tasks and situations; some of them even worked outside the home—at least, on a part-time basis. Nancy was overwhelmed with the responsibility of keeping three young children healthy and alive.

Nancy's husband tried to be helpful when he told her about his secretary at work and her great skill at multitasking. All Nancy had to do was maintain concentration on simultaneously occurring events. Neither cleaning, nor cooking, nor even supervising the children would take her undivided attention at every moment. Keeping an eye on some of the other activities or events while she was engaged in a different one would enable her to be on top of things. Nancy tried to follow her husband's advice but her frustration increased.

Her self-esteem plummeted when she compared herself to her husband's secretary and the other young women in their community. They were able to take things in stride. They made time for visits to the day-spa or to the massage therapist. They chauffeured their children to different events and cooked nutritious meals. To make things worse, Nancy knew that her mother had raised five children and here she had difficulty keeping up with three. In her own mind, wherever she looked, Nancy did not measure up. Her low self-esteem kept her from talking openly to the women in her community and rendered her emotionally isolated. Nancy's interest in sexual activities vanished.

Before multitasking became a characteristic aspired to, investigators, concerned with various aspects of attention, described attention as the sharp edge of consciousness and the process of recognition in action (McCrone, 1993), thus linking attention and recognition (matching information to already stored information in the brain) as two parts of the same focusing process within the brain. But attention selects and draws into the foreground specific aspects of the surroundings, while other actions may go on in the background that are ignored by the individual. Although some believe that it is possible to attend simultaneously to several events, what actually occurs is that the individual's mind must shift back and forth between stimuli, which causes attention to oscillate and which creates fatigue. These random, energy-wasting shifts in attention can be prevented through strengthening concentration—the very thing women, for the sake of the family, are not a allowing themselves to indulge in.

In her book *Composing a Life,* Mary Catherine Bateson (1989) seemed to ascribe gender-related characteristics to attention. Based on her observations, she explained men's way of attending as purpose-related and having a narrower focus than women's way of attending which is broader in focus and responding and adapting in nature. As basis for her thoughts she used personal experiences, such as her husband's not discontinuing his activities and focus at times that she was interrupting him. She, on the other hand, automatically dropped whatever she was doing in order to respond to his interruptions.

Rather than assuming that attention skills are genetically linked to gender, Bateson's description would indicate that women are trained through their roles in life to be able to attend simultaneously to several different stimuli. A woman attending to the family meal or the laundry will drop everything at the sound of a crying baby in the house. It is also the woman who answers most of the family phone calls, and—for her convenience—in the average home there is usually a telephone installed in the kitchen. Other family members may demonstrate a hearing impairment for the sound of a ringing phone but not so for the spoken statement "It is for you." As women are expected to attend to many minor crises, they have come to accept and adapt to these demands on their attention (Maass, 2000).

Self-Focused Attention

A type of attention, self-focused attention, has been described as one of the moderator variables in psychological strategies for protecting one's self-concept (Campbell & Sedikides, 1999). As attention is directed inward, individuals are in a state of self-focused attention and become aware of the discrepancy between who they think they are (actual self) and who they would want to be (ideal self), or who they think they should be (ought self). Accepting the value of self-focused attention in strategies for enhancing individuals' self-concept, it is important to recognize that for many women self-focused attention can be of a negative nature, as discussed earlier in Chapter 3. Perhaps the emphasis on the negative aspects of their self-concepts prompts women to turn their attention to others' well-being rather than their own.

Tina: Response-Related Attention

Tina, the mother of three small children, found it impossible to avail herself of periods of time where she could focus on her own interests. Even when the children were taking their naps, she used that time for cleaning and doing laundry. Her marriage was deteriorating. She was exhausted at the end of the day, regarding her husband's attempts at sex as just another chore to perform. Separation was a consequence and a learning experience for Tina.

While her children were on their scheduled visitations with their father during the separation, Tina fabricated reasons for going over to the house to check on the children. Being by herself without the need for constant alertness and vigilance regarding her children's well-being, she felt lost and almost paralyzed in their absence. The family is reunited now and Tina has learned that she does not have to jump in and make peace whenever the children are arguing among themselves. Not every episode of crying needs her immediate attention. Now she is able to set aside some time to focus on her own interests, such as writing. At the same time the children have the opportunity to learn how to resolve their little conflicts, resulting in closer bonding among the siblings and increased feelings of competence for all. And yes, Tina's interest in sex is increasing.

Whether we call it multitasking or response-related attention skills or lack of self-focused attention, this trait is one of many that might develop during women's transformation into wives which, as Heyn (1997) pointed out, can be detrimental to their happiness.

5
Symptom Manifestation Within Relationships

The list of factors contributing to women's reduced sexual desire is long. In addition to physical, cultural, and psychological factors, interpersonal aspects, such as partnership duration (Klusmann, 2002) and spousal dissatisfaction (Shokrollahi, Mirmohamadi, Mehrabi, & Babaei, 1999), have an impact on the individual's sexual interest and sexual responses.

The many ways developmental influences affect women's attitudes in the search for their identity and their role in future relationships were explored in the previous chapter. How do these influences become determining factors within intimate relationships? Lack of attention to key features in the differences between male sexual responses and female sexual responses has slowed general understanding of how gender differences in sexual responses impact female sexuality within a given relationship. It is most often the woman's wish for intimacy that prompts her sexual response. With that, desire and arousal bring emotional and physical satisfaction with or without orgasm. By comparison, a need for intimacy is often not of the utmost importance in the male sexual response cycle, whereas orgasm usually is. Thus, if the wish for intimacy does not find fulfillment in a sexual relationship, the woman's sexual desire may plummet.

Emotional Emptiness and Sexual Desire

Although in many instances, the emotional or psychological factors instrumental in the lack of sexual desire can be found in current relationships that a woman is involved in, some women coming from an unemotional family background may leave sexuality an unexplored domain of their lives. Emotionality and sensitivity are discouraged, while practicality, logic, and absence of sentimentality are encouraged in the growing-up experience. Emotionality serves no purpose; it is not needed.

Joan: Sex on Schedule

Joan and Fred have been married for almost 15 years and have struggled with adjusting to each other's sexual needs for several years. Joan cannot remember ever having experienced desire for sexual activities. She believes her poor self-esteem is the reason for her lack of desire. She grew up in an unemotional family environment where she was never praised for what she did right but rather criticized for what she did wrong. Because she was an only child, she had no opportunity for comparison; would her parents have treated any siblings the same way or was it truly her incompetence? During her developmental years Joan never found the answer to that question.

Encouraged by her parents and as an act of self-protection, she repressed most emotions within her. As long as she didn't feel it, it would not disturb her, was her reasoning. Her marriage to an emotionally unexpressive man did not require Joan to develop any sensitivity for her feelings. In fact, the marriage seemed like a logical continuation of her childhood and adolescence lived at her parents' home.

In the absence of warm and passionate feelings, Joan needed to adjust to her husband's wishes for sex. They lived in Alaska at the time they reached a solution that seemed to work for them. Fred worked for a shipping company, and his work schedule included occasional trips with overnight stays, but he could count on being home for weekends. If they had sexual activities once a week on the same day, Joan would be able to prepare herself mentally for it and—even more important—she did not have to worry about it the rest of the time. Fred liked the security of knowing that his needs would be met. This arrangement also relieved him of trying to figure out what would put Joan in the mood for sex; she took care of it herself.

Although Joan did not feel desire for sex, she did not develop an aversion to it because she felt she was in control. During their sexual activity Joan was at times able to become aroused to the point where she experienced orgasm, which pleased her husband and he could then focus on his own climax.

This arrangement may not work for couples who would prefer more emotional or spontaneous involvement, but it appeared to be a solution that kept Joan and Fred relatively satisfied with their relationship. In effect it was a situation of exchange. Joan made a certain time on a regular schedule available for Fred in exchange for freedom from concerns about sex for the rest of the time. Fred, on the other hand, was assured to get his opportunity for sex without having to plan on how to seduce Joan. In sex "barter works only when it is done openly and neither party feels coerced" (Hajcak & Garwood, 1987, p. 110); and Joan and Fred functioned well on this basis. Their arrangement was successful in reducing significant pressures related to sex, and they were able to reinstate it after they returned to their home state after their daughter's birth.

Shifts in Sexual Attitudes and Behavior

As television, movies, and magazines seem to reflect a shift to more liberal sexual attitudes and behaviors, questions about the magnitude of this change especially as it involves the female population arise. Has a progression of liberal sexual attitudes continued ever since the "sexual revolution," or have we observed a recent turn to a more conservative stance? As was discussed in Chapter 4, there are many influences at work when girls and young women struggle with shaping their own identity as women as well as sexual beings. Do the young girls and women of today share the same sexual values and behaviors of their sisters of about 40 years ago? It would seem reasonable to assume that changes in society, such as high divorce rates and increases in AIDS cases, would have an impact on the sexuality of young people.

Karen: From Sexual Promiscuity to Health Obsessions

When Conrad and Karen sought marriage counseling, their current unhappy situation seemed to have been a direct consequence of the liberal sexual attitudes they had subscribed to in the past. Karen, having been raised in a strict, devout Catholic family, succumbed to the seduction and promises of the sexual revolution. In the early 1970s she had lived a promiscuous life, telling herself that it would be good to have as much sexual experience with many different partners as possible before settling down to start a family.

Before Karen and Conrad met they both had contracted genital herpes, a condition that hardly raised an eyebrow at the time because it had become so common among young people. It certainly was not bad enough to preclude motherhood, and Karen delivered the couple's twin girls by Caesarean section—a small price to pay.

Raising her children prompted Karen's mental and emotional return to the values of her family of origin. The sight of her little daughters filled her with a mixture of emotions: gratitude, guilt, and anxiety. She was grateful for their apparent health, but experienced strong guilt feelings about her past sexual behaviors. Anxiety was brought on by the slightest physical symptom of illness or discomfort in both herself and her daughters. A runny nose or a slight cough threw Karen into high states of anxiety.

Stories in the media of the increasing number of AIDS cases made Karen fear that she might have unknowingly contracted the disease during her earlier time of promiscuity. Windows of 5 to 10 years of latent infection could mean that she had the deadly virus and might have passed it on to her children. Although Karen would have preferred to breastfeed her daughters, she decided not to even though tests and frequent visits to the doctor's office did not indicate any reason not to nurse her daughters.

Karen's anxiety and preoccupation with health issues overshadowed the family life. Any happy occasion, such as the girls' birthdays or their successful passing of developmental milestones or Karen's and Conrad's wedding anniversary, brought up Karen's underlying questions, How long is this good time going to last? When will I be safe in knowing that I did not contract the AIDS virus? With all this gloom and doom the couple's sex life deteriorated until it was nonexistent. Sex to Karen became a constant reminder of her sinful past and the guilt of possibly having damaged her own and her children's health. Conrad did not share her guilt feelings and after some years could not tolerate the high level of anxiety so pervasive in the family atmosphere. Although he recognized the danger to his daughters that might be caused by Karen's overprotectiveness, he decided to leave the marriage.

How Are Changes in Attitude and Behavior Linked?

Questions in the area of social psychology may be, How are changes in attitudes linked to changes in behavior: does one cause the other or is there no relationship between the two? We can find an array of different answers in the relevant literature. Some theorists propose that attitudes develop in response to situations, perhaps as an attempt to reduce cognitive dissonance (Kleinke, 1978), whereas other investigators report significant correlations between sexual attitudes and behaviors (DeLamater & MacCorquodale, 1979), indicating that behaviors follow attitude change (Bentler & Speckart, 1979) or that attitudes and behaviors may change at the same time or in some reciprocal manner (Kelman, 1974).

Paradoxically, a Planned Parenthood (2001) report related that almost half of sexually active, unmarried adolescents believed that premarital sex was not acceptable under any circumstances. In other words, even while they were engaged in premarital sex, they were also convinced that it was not permissible. Thus, one can find support for all kinds of possibilities in the literature. Increases in permissive sexual attitudes and changes in sexual behaviors have been most pronounced within the female population (Ciabattari, 2001; Rubin, 1990). In a review of several national surveys it was found that for the time period between 1970 and 1988, young males aged 15 to 19 years showed only slight increases in premarital intercourse activities, while for young women of that age group sexual intercourse doubled (Seidman & Rieder, 1994).

In a recent cross-temporal meta-analysis Wells and Twenge (2005) examined 530 studies with a population of 269,649 young individuals and found that although both young men and young women became increasingly more active sexually in the years between 1943 and 1999, the largest shifts were observed among girls and young women. The age of first sexual intercourse had decreased from 19 to 15 years among young women and the percentage of sexually active young women increased from 13% to 47%. Approval of premarital intercourse increased from 12% to 73% among young women and from 40% to 79% among young men while feelings of guilt about sexuality decreased.

Observing that the correlation between attitudes and behaviors appeared stronger among the population of young women, the investigators took their data to support theories that proposed a larger cultural effect on women's sexuality than on men's. If we accept the investigators' explanation that these findings indicate women's greater vulnerability in attitudinal and behavioral changes to cultural influences, can we perhaps generalize within the area of women's sexual desire that young women become more accustomed to sexual interactions—at least, premaritally—even if they don't always enjoy them?

And consider another hypothesis: With the earlier onset of women's sexual intercourse during the last several decades, could it be expected that their interest in these sexual activities would vanish earlier, especially when confronted with the many stresses of daily life? With an earlier start, women may have as much as five decades or more to be sexually active. Will this prolonged period lead to increased sexual excitement through practice or to increased boredom because everything has been tried already?

Rhonda: Changing Priorities

Rhonda remembers the fall of 1969 as a turning point in her life. She was 18 years old and her parents packed her off to college a few states away from their hometown. Although she felt anxious about leaving home for the first time in her life, there was also a certain curiosity and a sense of adventure mingled in with the anxiety. Once settled in her new environment, she adjusted well to the dormitory life and made many friends. She took her studies seriously but there was still time for fun and play. Her new friends were instrumental in introducing her to a range of extracurricular activities; in addition, there seemed to be a plethora of young men to date. On most of her dates she easily became aroused sexually and enjoyed her newly discovered sexuality.

During the summer preceding their move to different colleges, Rhonda and her high-school boyfriend had decided to become sexually intimate, perhaps as a vague promise to remain faithful to each other while away at college. The event of losing her virginity had not been as remarkable as Rhonda had anticipated. With high expectations and high anxiety coupled with inexperience on both sides, the event was over almost as soon as it began: the boyfriend's excitement about his first act of sexual intercourse, not surprisingly, resulted in his premature ejaculation. They tried a few more times but there was no great improvement in the quality of their lovemaking.

Rhonda was about to graduate from the nursing program when she met the man of her dreams. Tall, blond, elegant-looking Rob was in his final year of medical school. His deep, soft voice when he talked to her made Rhonda melt inside. He could be gentle but also very passionate. They fell deeply in love; their lovemaking was heavenly. Rhonda's good grades landed her a job as nurse in a local hospital, and although Rob still had a long way ahead of him before he would become a full-fledged physician, they decided to get married.

Although they now lived together, it seemed to Rhonda that they had less time to spend together than before their marriage. Both of their schedules were so hectic that they hardly saw each other for more than a few hours on any one day. When he was at home, Rob needed to study to keep up with the requirements for his career. Their lovemaking was still passionate but there was less time for planning a romantic setting or for lengthy foreplay. With the increasing amount of pressure about finishing his medical training, Rob seemed to become less attentive.

Toward the end of Rob's residency they decided to start a family. Rhonda delivered a baby boy and a baby girl within 18 months of one another. However, their financial situation required that she continue her job on a full-time basis. At the end of the day she sank into bed exhausted. If Rob was less attentive, she did not seem to notice, but when he initiated sexual activity she found herself less interested and less excited. After 6 years of marriage Rhonda asked herself what had happened to her passion? She still loved Rob, but the excitement she had felt in the beginning, the chemistry between them, had been eroded in less than 10 years' time. How did it all get lost in the daily grind of job, children, and household chores? Rhonda had not actually changed her basic values and beliefs about sex; the primary change became a behavioral change in the level of priority she and perhaps Rob assigned to sexual activities.

The Pressure for Orgasm

As a consequence of the more open discussion about female orgasms in the past decades, what should be a pleasurable occurrence has become a point of increased pressure for many. Various aspects of the impact of the pressure for orgasm on female sexual desire in heterosexual unions are described in other parts of the book. Often women who feel misunderstood by the men in their relationships may expect that other women would have more empathy and understanding because they as women would be able to realize that orgasms—while great to experience—do not constitute the whole sexual relationship.

Although these women may not want to enter a lesbian relationship, the general assumption that women understand women better than men do can be convincing. Yet some women are just as obsessed as men about their female partners' orgasm.

Kim and Lucy: The All-Important Orgasm

When Kim and Lucy came for their first therapy session it was very obvious that Kim felt extremely uncomfortable. Although the appointment was scheduled in Kim's name, it was Lucy who had arranged it. The presenting problem was stated as inability to achieve orgasm. Lucy acted as the spokesperson, stating that Kim had never experienced an orgasm either in her marriage or in their relationship. As Lucy continued to talk, Kim was squirming in her chair and one could see that she would have preferred to be anywhere else but where she was.

Kim, the mother of a young daughter, had been married for about 10 years when her husband filed for divorce. The reason was sexual incompatibility. For as long as Kim could remember, her libido had been low. Although she had engaged in some romantic fantasies like most girls her age, she never felt physically aroused and she never masturbated. She liked her husband Larry and marriage seemed the thing to do. Initially, she did not dislike sex; it felt rather pleasant, even though she did not experience the big explosion people talked about.

Over time Larry became concerned about Kim's inability to become sexually aroused to the point of orgasm. He kept asking her during sex if she felt close to it and what she would like him to do. He made her orgasm his business. The more he pressured her, the less likely it became that Kim's level of arousal would increase. In fact, she was unable to relax and enjoy the touching and kissing as she had been able to in the past because she anticipated Larry's questions with such anxiety. Kim felt inadequate; she did not measure up to the average woman. What sexual interest she had experienced in the beginning of their relationship evaporated into nothing. More and more she dreaded their sexual activity and finally she refused to participate.

Ultimately, she and Larry divorced, following which Kim was involved in a few brief relationships; but her self-esteem had been so reduced during her marriage that she could not relax in any relationship with a man. She stopped dating and spent all her efforts on her job and raising her daughter. Through a friend at work she met Lucy. She liked Lucy, and they had several interests in common. They decided to move in together. Kim confided that she had never experienced an orgasm. Unfortunately, Lucy accepted that as a challenge. In their lovemaking Lucy worked hard to bring Kim to the point of orgasm, but without success.

As Lucy related the story, she sounded exasperated. The therapist inquired about the length of their relationship. Lucy answered, "Three weeks," and Kim corrected her, "Less than that, just a little over two weeks." Asked how Kim felt in this new relationship, she burst out, "It's just as much pressure as my marriage was. Lucy is very attentive to me and I really like that. But when I fail to perform, I experience the same anxiety and self-doubt that I had gone through in my marriage. I wish people would stop pressuring me and leave me alone so I can enjoy at least some part of sex. But no, it's always orgasm, orgasm, orgasm!"

Shocked over Kim's outburst, Lucy started to cry. The therapist attempted to put the situation into perspective: it was a very short time that the two women had known each other, and it might be easier for both of them to slow down the speed with which they had tried to develop the relationship. Kim agreed with that. For the first time in the session she seemed to feel more comfortable. However, Lucy was reluctant to continue their relationship on a less intensive level. She stated her feelings were hurt and she did not know if she could forget Kim's complaints.

Kim and Lucy's short relationship did not survive this eruption. They had not known each other long enough to be able to trust and consider the other's point of view. Kim called to cancel their tentatively scheduled next appointment, stating that Lucy had moved out as soon as they left the therapist's office. Kim sounded relieved and managed to ask if it would be agreeable if she called for another appointment in the future because she realized that there may be ways of working on improving her sexual desire as well as improving her overall self-concept.

Effects of Sexual Compliance on Sexual Desire

As the level of sexual desire varies from person to person and even within the same person at different times, two partners who love each other and decide to share their lives may find out that they are not perfectly matched with regard to sexual desire. Furthermore, much has been said about the differences between men and women along this dimension. What are people to do when they have entered a committed relationship only to find out that their sexual interests are not compatible? It is a situation fraught with conflict.

People in love with each other will try hard to avoid or minimize the conflict. They may compromise by putting the other partner's desire above their own and willingly participate in sexual activities that they originally had not wanted to engage in. Professionals in the field of sex research have referred to this situation as "sexual compliance" or "consensual unwanted sex" (Impett & Peplau, 2002; O'Sullivan & Allgeier, 1998). Both men and women at times will agree to engage in sexual activity that they do not actually desire; however, in general, women are more often the compliant partners.

Based on current research findings, men are more likely than women to initiate sex, not only in new relationships, but also in ongoing dating and marital relationships (Impett & Peplau, 2003). Therefore, women most frequently are put in the position where they either participate in sex because they desire to do so or because they are compliant with their partners' wishes—or they may refuse. In a study of married couples, participants were asked about their responses to their partners' wishes for sex at times that they themselves do not feel sexually interested (Carlson, 1976). Of the wives, 84% stated that they usually participated in the sexual activity, whereas only 64% of the husbands reported that they were compliant.

Researchers have listed many reasons for women's greater compliance with undesired sex: Beliefs about "uncontrollable" male sexuality may influence some women to think that the man is too aroused to stop and that it is useless or unreasonable not to comply (Gilbert & Walker, 1999). Or they fear that the man will look for and find more willing female partners because of his strong sex drive (Impett & Peplau, 2000). The influence of traditional gender roles, such as women needing to satisfy a partner's needs in order to maintain intimacy (Impett & Peplau, 2002; O'Sullivan & Allgeier, 1998), constitutes a different kind of reasoning along relational or partner-centered lines. Reviewing the research literature, DeLamater (1987) concluded that women in their relational orientation tend to view sexuality as an integral part of an ongoing emotional relationship, a conclusion that is not always confirmed in reality.

Another reason for women's greater compliance rates can be found in the gender differences in power (Muehlenhard & Schrag, 1991). Although many contemporary couples accept and practice equality in their relationships, there is still a substantial minority of relationships where the husband holds greater power than the wife (Blumstein & Schwartz, 1983). Power and situations of dependence can have strong impact on female sexuality, as will be explored in more detail in Chapter 6.

While the reasons for women's sexual compliance are significant and varied, the consequences often are quite similar. Sexual compliance coming from loving feelings early in a relationship may bring a sense of accomplishment to the woman because of the importance of accommodating a loved partner. However, as the relationship grows older and more filled with other responsibilities, the same woman could become disenchanted or even resentful.

In relationships where the woman has not communicated any overt displeasure this could become problematic. According to popular opinion, a woman's hesitancy to refuse sex has been interpreted as uncertainty about her intentions and has been linked to rape (Shotland & Hunter, 1995). The male partner in the relationship may interpret any slight hesitancy on the woman's part which is then followed by compliance as part of the sexual game plan: for example, "women say no when they mean maybe, and they say maybe when they mean yes."

The male partner convinced of the truth of his assumption will most likely become more persistent in his initiation of sex, expecting his female partner's compliance after initially having played "hard to get." While he is persisting in his pursuit—not knowing exactly what is going on in her—she will become annoyed and indignant because her wishes are discounted. With those feelings and thoughts impacting her, her interest in sexual activities will take a nosedive. Over time, sexual compliance may turn into sexual avoidance.

Carol: Whispering No

Carol had married the love of her life. Peter was everything she had ever dreamed of in a man. How could she be so lucky that he chose her for his bride? For the most part, their sexual life was sheer ecstasy, except sometimes when Carol came home from her job tired. However, it did not take Peter long to convince her that she was not too tired for sex.

After the birth of their two children Carol was tired more often. She had cut down her working hours to half-time, but it became more and more difficult to find a few minutes to rest before facing dinner preparation and childcare. Carol tried to avoid sex a few times by quietly going to bed and dozing off to sleep. Peter, however, aroused her from her light sleep, trying to make love. Hesitating, in her low voice Carol would try to make some excuses, but Peter did not seem to hear them. Did he not hear her or did he not take her seriously? Carol wondered.

Finally, one night Carol exploded. She had been anxious as well as tired. Her anxiety stemmed in part from her work and also from wondering if she could get to sleep without having sex. Over the years her sexual desire had declined, and Peter had made some remarks about Carol "losing her spark." As usual, Peter initiated sex. Carol pleaded, "No, please not tonight; I am too tired." Peter's "Come on, Honey, you'll enjoy it—you always do," sent her straight out of bed. As she ran out of the bedroom she screamed, "Can't you get it through your thick head, I am not always in the mood for sex. For years I have tried to make you understand that I don't want to have sex as often as you do, but you always go ahead with it anyway."

Carol's outburst took Peter by surprise. He thought Carol's meekly voiced no's meant that she wanted him to pursue her more ardently. Now his feelings were hurt and he promised her he would not touch her ever again unless she begged him on her knees. The next morning Carol tried to explain how she had tried to let him know without hurting his feelings and hoping that he would understand that she at times was not in the mood for sex. For several weeks they did not talk to each other except for the communication necessary to maintain the family's functioning.

They decided to try marriage counseling. It took a while to rebuild the emotional closeness they had once experienced. Peter claimed that he could not trust Carol to be honest with him, and Carol thought she could not trust Peter to accept and honor her wishes. Over the years they had chipped away at the trust they had had in each other in the past. Carol's reluctance to voice clearly her wishes not to have sex when she was tired paved the way for the erosion of their mutual trust. Her outburst—when she thought she could not take it anymore—made Peter feel that he had been made a fool of for years.

Peter realized that he had not listened well and acted mostly on his assumptions of what Carol wanted. Carol learned to communicate more clearly and openly. What were her intentions when she decided not to express herself clearly because she did not want to hurt Peter's feelings? Did it mean that she was afraid to take a stand for what she liked and did not like? Was she afraid that Peter would love her less or leave her if he knew she wasn't always in the mood for sex? Whatever the underlying reasons for not wanting to hurt Peter's feelings were, Carol was hurting her own feelings for her husband.

When Carol and Peter finally resumed sexual activities, their lovemaking was far from the spontaneous and passionate encounters of their past. Both had to overcome a certain degree of awkwardness, and there were occasions where misunderstandings prevented them from enjoying an exciting sexual encounter. Carol, in particular, experienced a variation in her sexual interest. At first, with the threat of losing Peter, she had become more desirous of sex with him while he was still hesitating to let passion overwhelm him. Then her desire, which had been reduced prior to their confrontation, remained at a lower level for a while.

It would not be expected that Carol's level of sexual interest would match the desire she had felt years ago at the beginning of their relationship. She realized the need for increasing her sexual interest by not letting her daily activities overwhelm her to the point where she was too tired for lovemaking and by preparing herself with romantic literature or music to rekindle her passion.

Some interesting questions arise considering Carol and Peter's situation: Did he really not know that Carol was not always interested in sex or did he know and pursue her anyway because he wanted to have sex despite her reluctance? Or did he believe that he could get her aroused enough so that she would not feel as tired once they got started? These questions were not addressed by either Carol or Peter.

Sexual Sacrifice

O'Sullivan and Allgeier (1998) in a study of college students in dating relationships found that many participants had been aware that their partners at times had little interest in a sexual encounter but had consented to unwanted sex. For the interested partner it is important to know how the uninterested partner feels about his or her sexual sacrifice (i.e., engaging in sex even though desire is low or lacking). At the same time it is also important for the uninterested partner to understand the feelings of the partner who wants sex and goes ahead with it despite being aware of the other's sacrifice.

When this issue was explored recently with students in a college Human Sexuality class the following reasons for engaging in sexual intercourse even though not feeling much desire were given by female responders (listed in the order of frequency of response): "To make my partner happy." "In order to avoid a fight or argument." "I was afraid not to." How did the young women feel when they engaged in sexual intercourse even though they were not interested? Again, answers are ordered according to frequency: "I felt bored, just wanted it to be over" (by far the most frequent answer). "All I wanted to do is sleep." "I felt like I was being used, like someone to help him achieve orgasm." "I did it because my partner does it for me at times."

Several of the young women thought that their partner had not been aware of their lack of desire, mainly because they thought their partners only cared about their own wants and wishes. A few women assumed that their partner was—at least, at times—aware of their low desire but that they did not seem to worry much about it, either because they reciprocated at other times or because they simply did not care. With one exception the women admitted that they would engage in sex again under the same circumstances and for the same reasons. Few had been in a position to initiate sex with a partner when they knew that partner did not share their interest at the time.

When asked about having sex with a female partner who might not have been interested at the time, the male students' responses fell into two categories: "I did not want to coerce her, but she eventually went along with it. I guess she enjoyed it," and "If she was not ready for it but did it anyway it's because she cares about me." They also thought that they would not act differently in similar situations in the future.

None of the students responding was married; a few were cohabiting, but most were single, living alone. Of course, this exploration of the students' opinions does not carry the weight of a controlled experiment with randomized populations. It merely constitutes an informal inquiry addressing a small sample of young people about their attitudes concerning this topic.

Impett and Peplau (2003) raised the question of whether the recognition of a partner's participation in sexual activity despite low desire enhances the level of commitment to the relationship. They suggested that it is necessary to consider the sexual motives of both partners in order to know the impact of sexual sacrifice on a relationship. In situations where one partner seeks sex for self-focused reasons without much concern for the other partner's motives for compliance, sexual sacrifice may not do much to stabilize the emotional balance and commitment in the relationship.

On the other hand, if sexual compliance can be understood within the framework of exchange theory, partners have opportunities for reciprocating; and compliant partners may find occasions when they receive special considerations from their partners at other times or in another area of the relationship (Lawrance & Byers, 1995). Even though people might hesitate to think about intimate relationships in terms of an exchange, they do take turns doing something special for their partner and reciprocate with kindness toward each other. Unless there is some give and take, feelings of resentment and bitterness will develop when one partner receives most of the benefits in a relationship.

For the few female students who reported participating in sex despite a lack of interest but because their partners reciprocated at other times, considering their compliance in exchange terms would seem reasonable. But for those women who engaged in sex without feeling desire and without reciprocity and who admitted that they would repeat their actions in similar situations, the question arises, How long can they continue with this behavior before they have exterminated any sexual desire they may once have felt? Impett and Peplau (2003) remind us that the Oprah Winfrey television show in 2001 devoted two episodes to the topic that millions of American women seem to have lost or extinguished their sexual desire.

"Turn-Offs"

Helen Singer Kaplan (1979), based on her work with patients who complained of inhibited sexual desire, proposed the hypothesis that their sexual desire is low not because it does not arise but because they have learned to "turn it off," most often at the moment when the first erotic sensations are felt or anticipated. Usually, the individual is not aware of the suppression because the "turn-off" occurs so rapidly and automatically, leaving the individual with no insight into the mechanism. On some level these individuals do not want or refuse to feel sexual. There may be many different reasons for the "turn-off" mechanism to spring into action.

Disappointments, anger, and resentment all can function very efficiently as "turn-offs." However, in our culture, slightly different factors seem to be linked with inhibition of sexual desire in males and females. More women than men may be "turned off" if they are angry with their partner. It is more common for women to lose their desire for sex with their partner when they feel hostile. Men can still feel a strong desire for sex with the partner they are angry at.

Constructing Walls of Anger

Anger and resentment are forceful agents in the deterioration of relationships. When partners experience emotional pain that they attribute to behaviors in the other, they often perceive their anger as some sort of protection—protection from being hurt again. The anger seems to strengthen their resolve not to become soft or forgiving in their attitudes toward the partner. They build their wall of anger around them over many years, brick by brick. Every time they feel disappointed, rejected, or being taken advantage of by the partner, there goes another brick.

Although both male and female partners are capable of constructing walls of anger, this tendency seems to be more prominent in women. Perhaps because of a general condition of helplessness that women have experienced over generations due to the inequality in their social and economical standing, open expression of perceived injustices and demands for resolution have not been available options for many women. Thus, the smoldering anger has become a wall behind which to retreat. When one is in the emotional grip of anger and resentment that have been built up over time, it is difficult to engage in erotic fantasy. In fact, that might be the very thing to avoid because it could lead to weakening and crumbling of the wall of anger.

Claire: Charity Sex

Claire and Gus have been married for about 16 years and they have two children. Although they began their marriage as a loving couple, Claire soon found out that Gus, as the only son in a family with three daughters, was quite spoiled. Gus was a hard-working young man, but he entered marriage in the same carefree manner that he had enjoyed when he lived with his family of origin.

Claire, also holding outside employment, expected help around the house from Gus, especially after the children were born. When Gus "forgot" to do some of the chores, Claire silently completed them but not without building up resentment over the years. It was difficult enough for her to keep the house looking decent with being out on her job and taking care of the children. The least Gus could do was take care of his personal items, she thought.

When Gus was in the mood for making love, Claire often was tired and resisted or she gave in reluctantly. In response, Gus developed a passive-aggressive attitude, which increased his "forgetfulness." If Claire complained, he reminded her that even if he helped around the house, she still refused to have sex with him. She countered with stating that Gus sat down in front of the TV and became absorbed in it for hours. Claire did not interrupt his TV watching; after completing the chores and seeing to it that the children were getting ready for bed, she quietly went to bed herself—sometimes pretending to be asleep when Gus entered the bedroom.

When he returned home from work, Gus found himself becoming depressed and angry more days than not. By now both spouses interpreted each other's behaviors in the worst ways without ever checking to find out what the other really meant. Finally, Gus mentioned the possibility of divorce if the situation did not change. He wanted to be loved and accepted, and he was tired of getting "charity sex" every once in a while. He suggested marriage counseling. After a few sessions that apparently were filled with scheduling problems on the therapist's side, they were on their own once again.

It is interesting to note that Gus was the one who suggested counseling and who after the first failed attempt at counseling located another therapy agency. He admitted that he still loved Claire; all he wanted was for her to show him affection. His anger over feeling rejected found its expression in sarcasm. Gus realized that it did not help him, but at the moment of his hurt, sarcastic remarks were all he could come up with.

Although Claire's resentment was still overwhelming any romantic feelings, she knew she did not want a divorce. Reminding Claire that sex is part of a marriage most likely would not have solved anything at this point. Claire needed to explore ways to make sex a desirable activity for her own reasons. Because women are only too ready to take on chores or caring for others as their own responsibility—whether they enjoy these activities or not—it is important to avoid any resemblance of sex to marital duty. The notion of marriage including a set of agreements can be introduced at a different point in the process.

In this marriage, as in so many others, communication was a significant problem area. Because Claire's stated reason for not wanting sex because of tiredness seemed to be connected with the fact that Gus did not take care to put his personal items in the proper place or forgot to complete a chore, Gus assumed that if he did remove the disturbing items or performed the chore, he was entitled to have sex with Claire. This link between her refusal to have sex and his forgetfulness made sex a commodity to be traded in their relationship, which—simply stated—meant to Gus, "Pick up my things one day, get sex in the evening."

Claire may have noticed the occasions when Gus demonstrated that he could remember to do better, but in her mind it did not elate her to the point of desiring sex at that moment. She was pleased that there was one less thing for her to do, but she did not make the connection to sexual activities. At best, she was not in a bad mood generally speaking; she might have enjoyed a talk with the children or reading a book.

Over the years, the anger she had piled up toward Gus prevented Claire from experiencing loving feelings for him. Gus requested sex; it was something he wanted. But why should she give him what he wanted when Claire did not get what she wanted? Every time Claire saw things around the house that Gus had forgotten to pick up, she felt he did not care about her wishes; so why should she care about his?

Men's Inexpressiveness

An interesting explanation about men's silence was offered by Pittman (1993). Unlike women, men don't feel loved because somebody talks to them; therefore, men don't need to verbalize their love. According to this view, silence indicates a higher level of acceptance. Between men, love means never having to say anything. Men "escape to the sanctuary of male silence, away from the anxious world of emotions, from female-imposed sensitivity to the state of people's mind and the nature of people's relationships" (p. 204).

If we consider silence to reflect an elevated level of acceptance, logically it would follow that the less a man verbalizes his feelings, the more deeply he loves the woman he is with; in reality, however, most people would hesitate to agree. Women build emotional closeness with physical *and* verbal expressions. For women, sex means emotional closeness that can be expressed through verbal communication; but for men, their traditional sexual style has afforded them the freedom to feel entitled to their sexual desires without having to communicate much about their emotions (Maass, 2006).

A man's silence does not necessarily convince a woman of the depth of his love or acceptance of her; more likely, it leaves her emotionally isolated and lonely. Moreover, it may even give her the impression that the man is only occupied with the satisfaction of his own physical needs without concern for his partner's wants. Indeed, the silence might confirm in the woman's mind her own fears of not being attractive or interesting enough to hold his attention beyond the sex act. And it is this silence that often leads to the interpretation of abuse in men's sexual behavior. It is only a small step from this silence to the "Sexual Abuse Thoughts" described in the Nobre and Pinto-Gouveia (2003) study mentioned in Chapter 9.

Interestingly, it has been suggested that male inexpressiveness is not related to gender—as has been assumed all along—but that its connection is really to power (Sattel, 1983). Our customs and language reflect the differential prestige that is given to men in our society. Men's appearance of acting out of impersonal and unemotional rationality is a way to exercise the power. "To remain cool and distant when challenged is a strategy for keeping the upper hand that through its inexpressiveness conveys an image of strength." Male inexpressiveness is not a matter of inarticulateness or a socialized inability to respond to the emotional needs of others. Men use their inexpressiveness to guard their own position. "To not say anything—is to say something very important indeed: that the battle we are engaged in is to be fought by my rules and when I choose to fight. . . . In general, male inexpressiveness emerges as an intentional manipulation of a situation when threats to the male position occur" (Sattel, p. 122).

Jane and Nancy: The Silent Treatment

Jane and Nancy were sisters-in-law who found it extremely difficult to communicate successfully with their husbands. They had joined an ongoing group workshop about taking control of one's life. Both felt that their husbands controlled them through withdrawal and silence. Whenever Nancy wanted to discuss issues that in her mind still needed resolution, Fred withdrew. One can withdraw from a situation physically, mentally, or emotionally. Fred chose to walk away physically. His older brother Tom had applied a similar method for years in his marriage to Jane.

Actually, both brothers had learned this coping method from their parents: men don't argue; they preserve their position through silence. When Jane, Tom's wife, did not comply with Tom's wishes and demands, she got the "silent treatment" from him. In contrast to Fred, Tom did not even leave the room; he just wouldn't talk. Tom's method seemed to work: Jane soon caved in; she could not endure the silent treatment. She would do whatever it took to have Tom talk to her again—even if she did not like what she was complying with.

Interestingly but not surprising, both couples had been in marriage counseling for a brief period of time, with both husbands complaining mainly about the sexual part of their marriage. Nancy's way of responding to Fred's avoidance of discussing issues she considered important was through sexual avoidance; she was not in the mood for sex for long periods of time. Perhaps in response to the sporadic nature of their sexual encounters, Fred had developed the problem of premature ejaculation during their few and far between sexual activities. Jane's way of coping with the anxiety caused by Tom's silence was to be physically accessible for sexual intercourse while remaining mentally and emotionally numb.

How did Jane explain Tom's silence to herself? Her interpretation was that she had done something to displease Tom; his silence was his punishment for her. In her own opinion, had she really been at fault in some way? Jane rarely checked the reality of her "faulty" behavior, mainly because she was more afraid of the consequences she imagined—Tom abandoning her—than of wanting to know if she really was to blame for some egregious error. When Tom stopped communicating, Jane, in her overwhelming anxiety, perceived herself as being "on probation" until Tom decided to talk again after she had redeemed herself in his eyes.

Strong feelings of anxiety that almost automatically appear within the individual as a frequently used coping mechanism are not conducive to the development of sexual interest and desire. In fact, anxiety destroys the relaxation that is needed to enjoy the sensuous experiences that can be part of sexual activity. Anxiety functions as a distracting force as the individual is constantly "on guard" to avoid or prepare for the next crisis that may come in the form of criticism or silence (Elliott & O'Donohue, 1997).

Returning to the situation of Nancy and Jane, their husbands would probably agree that in the sexual area of their lives, their wives were in control. Did Tom know the power of his "silent treatment?" Probably he did or he would not have continued to apply it; but he must have been unaware of the consequences or he would have chosen another strategy, one would think. And neither Nancy nor Fred was probably fully aware of the consequences of their power plays.

What did Jane and Nancy learn in their "control" workshop? They realized that they had been responding to their husbands' behaviors in ways similar to what Fred and Tom were doing—withdrawing physically and emotionally and in Jane's case mentally and emotionally while complying physically. It is rare for partners in a power struggle who use similar tactics to come to a satisfactory resolution. They just prolong the damaging dance of control and power indefinitely until separation and divorce seem to be the only way to end it.

Reduced Sexual Desire Versus Reduced Desirability

When women by themselves or with their partners seek treatment at a clinic for sexual dysfunction, most often the woman becomes the identified client and the presenting problem is stated as "lack of sexual desire." In cases where sexual desire has been present in the past but is now reduced or lacking altogether, various tests are performed in addition to recording the sexual history of the client. The implication is that there is something wrong with the woman that needs to be fixed. It is less common for a man to approach a treatment agency with the statement, "My partner has lost interest in having sex with me; what am I doing that makes me less desirable than in the past?"

Rachel and Paul: Losing Desirability

When Rachel and Paul got married sex was extremely enjoyable for both of them. Paul was a terrific lover and Rachel appreciated his emotionality and sensuousness. Paul was ready for sex at least once a day. Rachel spent much energy at pursuing her career and on some evenings she was tired and would have preferred not to have sex at all and certainly not to spend hours at it. Paul was less ambitious professionally; although he enjoyed his work, he seemed less "stressed out" than Rachel did sometimes. Rachel's efforts paid off, however; she received several significant promotions in a relatively short period of time.

When she became pregnant, Rachel realized that she needed to continue working full-time. Her salary was more than twice what Paul earned and her insurance benefits were so much better that Paul had dropped his insurance through his employer. Because of her income they were able to buy a comfortable and attractive house.

Paul did not seem to mind his wife's higher income—after all, she had a college degree and he did not. He helped around the house when Rachel made a list of chores for him to do. Paul liked expensive cars and he thought that with their combined incomes he should be able to buy a new car at least every other year. Rachel did not see the need for new cars; the car she drove was almost 10 years old and it served her well. Paul was disappointed and argued about her old-fashioned stinginess. "Why not enjoy the money we have?" he asked, to which Rachel replied, "We need to put money aside for the kids' college fund and for our own retirement."

By now Rachel was pregnant again and knew that she was going to give birth to twin girls. Paul's idea was to celebrate the birth of the twins with a new automobile; he thought that would give them a great start in life. Couldn't Rachel see him as the proudest father collecting his family at the hospital in a shiny brand-new car? Rachel could not see his side of the argument, and it did not take long for Paul to threaten, "I might as well leave, I don't count for anything around here." Reluctantly, Rachel gave in. Paul was happy and ready for making-up sex, Rachel did not feel in a loving mood but she went along.

It was Paul's opinion that after an argument sex was important as a clear signal that the argument was over. Rachel was reluctant because she knew that she had yielded against her better judgment. She also realized a similarity between Paul and her father, which scared her. Her father had repeatedly put money into "get-rich-quick schemes," which kept the family in dire straits as she was growing up.

At the time Rachel and Paul came to therapy the twins were almost 4 years old, and the automobile that marked their arrival on earth had not been the last new car their parents argued about. In fact, their battles about expenditures increased in frequency. Many of them followed the script of the earlier one. Paul became verbally unpleasant when his wishes did not meet with instant approval. Rachel more often than not gave in and Paul wanted to celebrate the end of their fight with sex. From time to time Rachel refused to engage in sex after one of their battles.

Her resentment toward Paul was mixed with anger toward herself because she knew that her actions were incongruent with her own values. She handled the family's finances, which Paul interpreted as her having all the control. Her family's financial security was important to her and repeatedly she had agreed to spend more money than was in their best interest. She began to worry about what might happen if she lost her job. She worked harder to make sure that her job was not in jeopardy. The anxiety from the worry combined with the resentment toward Paul and the anger toward herself took a toll on her overall mood.

If she wanted emotional support and a hug from Paul, he interpreted that to be an invitation to sex. Thus, she deprived herself of any opportunity for emotional comfort. She was happiest when spending time with her children. Although she reminded herself frequently that she loved Paul, her respect for him decreased and she found it more and more difficult to be interested in having sex with him.

While assuming the responsibility for her family's well-being, Rachel had not taken on the responsibility for keeping her love for her husband alive. Although she had tried a few times to let him know how her feelings were affected by some of their disagreements and his reactions to her efforts to put the family on a secure financial basis, she did not follow through on her own judgment, defeated by the sheer force of his arguments. In order to salvage her feelings for Paul, she would need to develop a more effective way of communicating with him. Although she understood the logic of it, she felt hampered by the risk that Paul might leave and her children would not have the benefit of growing up in an intact family.

As Paul continues to complain about the reduced frequency of their sexual interactions and the lower levels of desire he experiences from Rachel, will he come to ponder the question, What is it about me that seems to make me less desirable to my wife now than when we first started out together?

No matter how well matched couples appear to be or think they are, characteristics from both partners that vary in some aspects contribute to the mix in the relationship, and some of those aspects may not blend in a complementary way. There are opportunities for dissonance in the overall combination. Many of the facets of interactions between partners have their roots in individual values and beliefs that people have developed during their formative years and beyond. There are also many influences from the individuals' families of origin and the individuals' own personality characteristics that enter the overall picture.

As can be seen from Rachel's story, some of her fears about Paul's tendency to spend money came from past experiences in her family of origin. Although she was aware of those influences from the past and of the fact that she acted in opposition to her values, she did not take a stand for what she believed in. The fear that Paul might leave and that her children would be deprived of the daily presence of a father in their lives prompted her to abdicate control and hand the power over to Paul. The next chapter will provide a closer look at women's relationship to power.

6
Women's Relationships to Power

Power and control dynamics can be observed to operate along the cultural lines of authority and coercion found in the status differential between men and women. "Men learn that control is the essence of manhood: control in the board-room, on the playing field, and in the bedroom" (Cassell, 1984, p. 52). Power can become connected to many different areas of human interaction, but it remains essentially a tactical choice where to apply it. Power "is not intrinsic to human sexuality,... but an element within the sexual realm which achieves certain desired ends (for some)" (Kuypers, 1999a, p. 21).

Power and Gender

In the sexual arena, we usually think of a scenario where the male partner has the power because in most cultures, men are the holders of power. The concept of masculinity incorporates images of power. As pointed out by Kuypers (1999b) in the introduction to the book *Men and Power,* power is "the single concept that organizes the passions and actions of men as a gender" (p. 7). Those who hold power expect it to be unidirectional and to be used when the situation demands it. In the male image, power is awarded and glorified, whereas the lack of it is judged harshly. Power is synonymous with success; those in power are in control. "Many men live with the shame that they are not powerful enough" (Kuypers, 1999b, p. 7).

In contrast, recommendations for women's behavior found in masculine mythology are quite different: "A woman above all should show deference to a man. When it comes to any conflict, the prevalent demand of our culture is that the woman defer to the man, whether the issue concerns practical matters, such as where and how to live, or intimate matters, such as when to make love. The presence of deference as a value internalized by women sets the stage for sexual exploitation" (Rutter, 1989, p. 65).

As discussed in Chapter 5, masculinity and men's inexpressiveness are to be understood in the asymmetrical dominance given to males in our society rather than in contrast with femininity. Male dominance is demonstrated in the positions of formal and informal power occupied by men in society, and the differential prestige is expressed in our language and customs (Sattel, 1983).

Emotions Beneath the Power Struggle

Some believe that the driving forces behind power struggles originate in individuals' feelings and needs (Kurcinka, 2000). Are the emotions that fuel power struggles different for men and women? If we consider Kuypers' (1999b) assumptions, men's feelings that drive the power struggle appear to be fear of being shamed and occupying a position of insignificance within their sense of masculinity. Their need for power is based on the fear of being overpowered and dominated by those who hold more power than they do.

For women, it is the fear of being abandoned by the power holder and thereby separated from the power vested in the male. For the female depending on the male's power, abandonment and separation from that power can lead to feelings of personal insignificance, losses of various types, such as material losses, loss of status and position, and even a degree of deprivation. According to this view, for both men and women, the significant motivator in power struggles is fear.

While women are believed to value emotional intimacy and romance in their sexual relationships, for men, on the whole, sexual desire is associated more with the pursuit of casual sex and short-term relationships—often in addition to being in a long-term relationship, such as marriage. Marriage provides the scenario for the full development of power plays.

Many of the gender power plays—parallel and in addition to the overt picture—contain covert scenarios that unfold in the couples' bedrooms. Because both sides have opportunities to assert some type of power, the repercussions can take on a twisted and complicated character, often not completely recognized and understood by the players in the drama. With the passage of time, the players become firmly entrenched in their positions and devote increasingly more time and energy to the support of strategies that resemble war games rather than marital interactions.

Marian: Sex, the Great Manipulator

Marian, a young woman working full-time and attending college on a part-time basis, admitted to having manipulated every romantic relationship she had ever been involved in—with negative results. Although she considered herself a good and caring person, she had been aware of her control attempts for a long time. Whoever the significant man in her life was at the time, Marian wanted to control his activities and insisted on his being with her at all times. What did she offer in return? Sex, along with the threat that she would end the relationship (stop the sex) if he did not comply.

However, in her fear of being abandoned, very much like Jenny, the young woman described in Chapter 3, she often tried to find out what the men wanted in a perfect woman and then she worked hard to supply it. In her way, Marian made sex an item of exchange, in this instance, for absolute devotion. One is reminded of another barter situation (described in Chapter 5)—Claire's linking sex with her husband's performance of chores. As in many other cases, Marian's system of exchange did not work indefinitely. None of her relationships lasted; even her 15-year marriage finally failed mostly because of her controlling ways.

After repeated failures, why did Marian continue with her manipulations? Obviously, what she was most in control of was that the relationship would end when the man exited after repeated exposure to Marian's complaints and attempts to curtail his outside activities. Marian knew the reasons for her self-defeating behaviors: insecurity and fear of abandonment. For many years she combated those fears with sex, money, and threats of leaving—always with the result of being left. Had awareness of the reasons for her manipulative behaviors helped her to learn a lesson? She was currently dating several men with different characteristics, different professions, and different goals for a relationship. With each one of them Marian tried to be exactly the woman he was looking for—except for her controlling tactics. She was mentally exhausted from playing different roles, although she was employing many of the same techniques in each relationship.

Marian may not have known how to change her behaviors, but she was also afraid of giving them up. Because the men stayed with her for varying periods of time, she told herself that her approach was working—at least, better than anything else she could think of. Her reasoning was not unique; most people maintain behaviors that overall are self-defeating but are successful part of the time because they don't know what the alternative would bring.

Power Plays and Social Exchange Theories

Borrowing from models of social exchange theories, Balswick and Balswick (1995) proposed a democratic exchange model of marital power. In the social exchange model, power consists of three components: the bases of power (sources), the processes of power, and the outcomes of power. Various resources, such as money, social status, employment, physical attractiveness, talents, and skills, make up the power base. The interactions of the involved parties constitute the power processes. These interactions may be exemplified by assertiveness and persuasion. Finally, who makes important decisions and who gets what he or she wants represent the outcomes of the power process. How each partner uses his or her resources in the process of negotiations for what each wants in the relationship determines the outcomes.

For instance, men may interpret women's reluctance to engage in sex as control or bartering attempts and respond with their own control methods, such as deciding not to let themselves fall in love or to avoid making commitments. Thus, out of suspiciousness the hurtful dance of control and counter-control efforts is initiated, preventing the formation of a stable, mutually satisfying, and enriching alliance between a man and a woman.

Denise: Consequences of Attempting To Avoid Payment

For Denise, a young psychology student, the struggle started early. She reported how vulnerable she had been when she transferred from a Catholic school to public high school. She tried to adjust to the new environment but was not accepted by her new classmates until a good-looking popular male senior student asked her out for a date. Then everybody wanted to be her friend. It seemed that the boyfriend had the power to bestow popularity on her, a condition she thoroughly enjoyed.

Soon her new boyfriend pressured her with demands for sex and threatened her that he would go back to his previous girlfriend if Denise remained noncompliant. Despite his threat, Denise went to a party with him, hoping he would not demand sex. Her hopes had no basis in reality. After the party he took her for a ride out in the countryside and when she refused to participate in sexual activities, he told her to get out of the car and walk home. Because she could not imagine how she would be able to get home, Denise decided to have sex with him. During the rest of her high school years she never went on drives with anyone again, Denise emphatically explained.

Since that first sexual experience Denise stated that she had never been able to experience any sexual desire for any man, although when she told the story, she was engaged to be married soon. She reported that she could not relax because she had felt manipulated by her classmates who wanted to be her friends only after she had gained the attention of a popular senior male student. And she thought the young man had overpowered her by forcing her to choose between walking home or having sex with him. When he gave her the ultimatum about returning to his previous girlfriend she could have ended the relationship with him before she found herself threatened with being stranded in the countryside. But she was afraid that ending the relationship with him would have cost her the standing she now enjoyed among her new friends.

If anyone had asked the young man at the time, he would probably have said that Denise tried to manipulate him because she went to the party with him after he had issued the ultimatum. At the end of her story Denise made it a point to say that although she remained friends with her classmates throughout high school, not one of them was her friend now and she added that she had learned a lot from the experience—but had she? It sounded as if she was still blaming her former classmates for what happened to her as well as the young man she had dated. Certainly, they played their parts in the overall situation, but Denise was a participant as well—as is so often the case in power scenarios.

Whatever she may have learned, she still did not understand that she had placed herself in danger not only because she entered her boyfriend's car but, more importantly, because she did so after he had informed her of his intentions. She knew what his goal was and she chose to remain the target. What did she expect to gain—to maintain the degree of popularity among her peers that she had achieved by dating this popular boy? Yet she did not want to pay the price for it. Certainly the boyfriend's behavior was not gentlemanly when he threatened to abandon Denise out in the country if she refused to uphold her end of the bargain. But there was no indication in Denise's report that she ever recognized her own failed attempts at manipulating the boyfriend. Did she believe that the power of her beauty would strengthen her refusal to have sex with him?

One wonders how Denise is going to cope with the lack of sexual desire in her new relationship. Did she inform her fiancé about it? Is she going to blame the boyfriend from long ago for not desiring sex with her future husband? They are both ready to make a commitment for life—one would hope that honesty will be a part of that commitment.

The Seductive Power of Benevolent Sexism

In marriage and romantic relationships the social organization of love—as it is defined in contemporary culture, emphasizing emotions rather than practical aspects—reinforces men's power over women. Popular beliefs, such as that women have a greater need for heterosexual love than men, lead to a power disadvantage for women as they may desperately seek to fulfill this need. Men, believing in women's need for love, realize their own power position.

Furthermore, for different reasons, both may endorse the characterization of women as being adorable creatures who ought to be protected and whose love is required for man's completion. This argument is in line with the ideology of benevolent sexism, which is a subtle form of prejudice that hampers gender equality (Glick & Fiske, 2001). In contrast to hostile sexism, an adversarial view of gender relations in which women are portrayed as seeking to control men, benevolent sexism appears to be based on a chivalrous ideology, offering protection and affection to women who endorse conventional roles, thereby reinforcing women's conventional behaviors.

Megan: The Knight in Shining Armor

Megan thought she had found her knight in shining armor when Harold rescued her from the unwanted attention of two young men in the restaurant where she had stopped for a cup of coffee. He seemed to know exactly how to keep the two men at bay and assured Megan that she was safe to enjoy her coffee; he would see to it. He did not sit down at her table but returned to his table nearby. After paying the waiter, Harold remained seated at his table until Megan was ready to leave. He got up and, being closer to the door, opened it for her. As she passed him, Harold told her he would escort her to her car, so that she would not be bothered again by those two obnoxious men.

Harold made sure that Megan was safely seated in her car before he asked her if she visited the restaurant at other times and added that he would be honored if she would join him there next week at the same time. He did not ask for her name or phone number, just politely reminded her to lock her car door and walked over to his car.

Megan was very impressed with his behavior: he had just tried to protect her without making a pass at her; he did not even inquire about her name. On her way home she kept thinking about him; he seemed so chivalrous. It did not take long for her to hope that he would be at the restaurant next week. She indulged herself in romantic fantasies that included her new hero. And, of course, she went to the restaurant at the same time a week later. He saw her right away and walked to the door to greet her. A wonderful courtship developed. Megan felt safe and special with Harold, who proved to be a good lover. Megan's sexual desire for Harold was strong.

Harold had been married before, and he told Megan that his previous wife did not appreciate his way of making certain that she was safe. She had laughed at his attempts to protect her. Megan thought, How could any woman not love the adoration and protection of this wonderful man? There had to be something wrong with Harold's ex-wife.

Before they left for their honeymoon they had found a nice apartment—or rather, Harold had found it—it was convenient to both their workplaces. When they returned from their honeymoon Harold suggested that he drop off Megan at her job before driving to his workplace. At the end of the day he would pick her up and they would return home together. Megan liked the arrangement; she did not have to worry about city traffic or where to park her car. The result was that they spent all their free time together.

Megan's coworkers had a habit of going out together after work, perhaps once a week. Although they wanted to include Megan, she had to decline because Harold picked her up at her workplace every evening. Sometimes she was able to join them for lunch. She enjoyed their company and told Harold about it. A week or so later Harold appeared at Megan's workplace around lunchtime. She had already left but Harold waited until she returned. When she saw Harold's face, Megan immediately felt a pang of guilt. Here he had wanted to surprise her for lunch and she had gone with her coworkers instead. Harold did not hide his disappointment and she agreed that she had been inconsiderate—even though she had not known Harold's plans for lunch.

That evening Megan was not really in the mood for sex. The guilt feelings she had experienced earlier now seemed to have a tinge of anger to them. However, Harold wanted to have sex and Megan did not want to disappoint him twice on the same day. She thought drinking a little bit of wine might improve her mood. It worked and she was able to enjoy their lovemaking. She used this aid to lovemaking from time to time when her sexual desire was lacking. One is reminded here of Lenore (whose story appears in Chapter 4), who also had used alcohol to help her overcome her reluctance to have sex with her husband.

About a year and a half into their marriage Megan was offered a significant promotion in her career. Naturally, she was excited that her supervisors had noticed her hard work and competence. It turned out that her new position was in another branch office in a different part of town. Harold listened patiently to Megan's report of the promotion. After her excitement had simmered down, he told her that he was glad her employer had recognized Megan's value. However, it was too dangerous for Megan to drive to work in that part of town, and it was not possible for him to drop her off on his way to work. Changing the location of her work was just not a wise thing to do. Besides, did she forget that they had been talking about starting a family soon? The new position would not lend itself to having children as she would have to work full-time, while in her present job she might be able to scale down to part-time work. It would be in Megan's best interest, concluded Harold, not to accept the promotion.

Megan's colleagues could not understand her decision to pass up this great opportunity; neither could her supervisors who had encouraged the promotion. Suddenly she was considered to be less competent than she had appeared earlier. The assignments given to her now were of a less challenging nature and Megan found herself on a dead-end track in her career. In the evenings on their way home Megan complained to Harold about her boring job. The spark had gone from her job and from her marriage.

Harold continued to be protective of Megan. In time he was able to convince his employer that Megan would be a great worker for their company. He described her as a very diligent employee who followed instructions willingly and precisely. Megan was grateful for the change in jobs. She had experienced some difficulty being happy for her colleagues when they received promotions. In fact, she admitted to herself being envious of them. In her new job people respected her as Harold's wife. Her new coworkers did not invite her to join them for lunch because they assumed that she would spend lunch breaks with Harold.

Even though she went out to work every day, she became more and more isolated socially. When Megan became pregnant with their first child, Harold found an appropriate house for them in the suburbs. The drive to work was longer, but Megan did not need to worry because they were still able to commute together and drop their child off at a daycare agency on their way to work. Everything was under control.

After the birth of their second child Megan developed postpartum depression, which made it impossible for her to return to work. In time her depression subsided with the help of medication, but she began to experience severe anxiety attacks whenever she was driving her car, even on short trips to the supermarket. She explained her lack of sexual desire as a side effect of the antidepressant medication.

Megan's anxiety attacks were treated by her psychiatrist with an additional medication. Did Megan perceive a connection between Harold's protective behaviors and her own increasing loss of competence? Not at that time. A few years later, Harold's complaints about Megan's sexual apathy brought her to a clinic for sexual dysfunction.

Protection, disguised as adoration within the framework of beneficial sexism, can be just as confining as more blatant forms of restriction, especially when adoration and protection are combined in a power framework, as will be seen in the next section.

Power and Sexual Desire

In our society it is relatively common for a man's sexual attractiveness to be linked with his achievements and social status, both of which usually increase with age. In that context, characteristics that detract from women's sexual attractiveness—facial wrinkles and gray hair—become associated with power and status in men; it makes them look "distinguished." The pairings of powerful, older men and young, beautiful women reflect the double standard of aging as well as the seductiveness of power.

Initially, adoration and protection combined within a power framework can include seductive elements and thus facilitate sexual desire. Individuals might want to be close to a source of power, perhaps for the protection it can provide or for the sense of being special it can bestow upon the recipient for having been chosen by a powerful person. On the other hand, over time, the fear of abandonment may interfere with the enjoyment of the relationship, or the personal characteristics of the power holder may influence the nature of the power process to an undesirable degree, so that the other partner feels disappointed or disgusted instead of satisfied and happy in the relationship.

Power gives those who hold it control over relationships. To comprehend the dynamics in a controller-controllee relationship to its full extent, it is necessary to understand the personality patterns of all the people involved, not just that of the controlling person. Although the controlling person may control or even victimize the target person, usually this cannot happen without the active participation of the controlled person in the relationship.

What brings the controller and the controllee together and what keeps them together? The two seem to attract each other like magnets. At first, the controlled person might admire a sense of decisiveness, determination, or strength in the other, especially if it is a romantic relationship between female controllee and male controller. Although an element of control can often be detected early in the relationship, the controllee is often inclined to explain it away. Statements like, "He is so concerned for my well-being; it is really an expression of his love for me" are rationalizations that serve as justification when the controller insists on knowing where his female controllee is at every moment.

The Sexual Attraction of Borrowed Power

With the enjoyment of the special status that power affords those who have it, such as money, social position, and the special recognition of the person's importance, among other things, the woman chosen by a powerful man often finds the privileges inherent in the power exciting enough to be sexually attracted to the man. However, the excitement that comes from the sense of power felt by being close to a powerful man may be of short duration, as it is what psychiatrist Natalie Shainess (1984) called "borrowed power." Women believe that they can overcome their own helplessness by attaching themselves to a powerful male;

however, when the male's enchantment wanes he may use his power to abandon the woman without much cost or trouble to himself.

Take the case of Anita, a divorced young mother of twin sons and a member of a women's therapy group (see also Chapter 10): her beauty attracted the admiration of a rich and powerful man who eventually became her husband. A few years into their marriage Anita became bored and got involved in an extramarital affair. At that point Anita found out what her husband's power could do to harm her. In court, her husband's lawyer proved her to be an unfit mother, and her husband was awarded sole custody of their two children. Anita had to settle for supervised visitation with her sons. She was not awarded alimony, but instead was ordered to pay child support to her former husband (Maass, 2002).

Remembering Denise's story (discussed earlier), one can understand Anita's situation in terms of a borrowed power scenario. While an individual remains in the good graces of the power holder, the power bestows special status as well as providing protection from minor hassles and irritations in daily life as there may be people paid to smooth the way. But that freedom from hassles and the special status have a price tag attached: the person with the "borrowed" power becomes, at least in part, a possession of the power holder.

Beauty, Women's Path to Power

Physical attractiveness is one way for women to feel powerful. Their beauty can be a significant tool in the seduction and manipulation of men. The attention beautiful women receive from men can be sexually arousing to them, especially if it is combined with promises of fulfilled wishes. As mentioned above, attention and admiration also serve to increase the woman's self-esteem. They make her feel important—even more so when the admiration comes from a man with power. One could argue that the wish to be close to power is an evolutionary desire because women busy with raising offspring needed the protection of a male and the more powerful a man is, the more protection he is able to provide.

Women like Barbara Amiel, former political columnist for the *Sunday Times* and wife of Canadian-born Conrad Black, who had been inducted into England's House of Lords in 2001 and whose more recent fall from grace has been reported in the popular press, find power sexy (McDonald, 2004). As she explained in a *Chatelaine* article entitled, "Why Women Marry Up," power is sexy in its own right but also because it encourages the owner of the power to feel self-confident and it inspires a shiver of subservience in those who approach it. There has been some speculation that Barbara Amiel—following Conrad's reduction in power—might replace him, her fourth husband, with a newer version.

Caroline: Beauty Within the Confines of Borrowed Power

When Caroline looks at her wedding picture she has difficulty remembering herself as happy as she must have been when the picture was taken almost 40 years ago. Only a few months had passed between her high-school graduation and her wedding. The journal she kept in those years gives evidence of the excitement she felt when Larry, the only son of the wealthiest family in town, wanted to date her, beautiful but poor Caroline.

Originally, Caroline had hoped to be able to go away to college and become a teacher, but Larry was not inclined to wait. Caroline's mother stressed the advantages of a life beside Larry over the insecure future of a schoolteacher. Dating Larry was exciting; all her friends envied her, and when word got around that Larry was serious about her, Caroline was treated like a princess in her small southern hometown. Already she enjoyed special social status, which could only be expected to increase once she became Larry's wife.

Caroline had made herself the promise to remain a virgin to her wedding day. But again, Larry, a young man with a strong sex drive, was not inclined to wait. His parents were out of town for a weekend, and Larry took Caroline home with him. Larry's adoration of her beauty and the elegant surroundings of his home bestowed a special, fairy-tale-like glow on Caroline's first sexual experience. Lunch at the country club the next day stretched the excitement into evening and into another night of passionate lovemaking. The main reason for the relatively brief period between Caroline's graduation and her wedding was her pregnancy.

Once she was Larry's wife and the mother of their first son, life changed. She was expected to fulfill her role as a member of the town's most powerful family. Her parents-in-law decided what type of house the young couple would live in and how it should be furnished and decorated. Larry expected Caroline to be available for sex whenever he wanted it. Now that they were married, he did not have to invest as much time in seducing her as he had in his courting days. Caroline's passion waned, as she became more of a captive than an excited participant.

What disturbed Caroline most was the practice of oral-genital sex, or more specifically, fellatio. During the last weeks of her second pregnancy Larry had instructed her in performing fellatio on him. He insisted on fellatio as part of their repertoire of sexual activities, but Caroline was repulsed by the idea and she almost gagged just thinking about it. Because fellatio could become a part of sex at just about any time, her remaining interest in sex vanished. The experience of receiving and giving oral sex is considered by men to be an expression of their power, whereas women perceive both giving and receiving oral sex from the position of powerlessness (Kimmel, 2000). This statement accurately describes Caroline's position.

Larry was not a cruel man, but having grown up in the world of the privileged, he regarded Caroline as a token or possession to be used as he wanted—after all, he had paid a high price for her. He complained about her lack of enthusiasm and eventually he found more stimulating events during his business trips away from home—although that did not mean that he refrained from sexual activity with Caroline.

To the outside world, Caroline's life was all a young woman could want. She had given birth to three wonderful healthy children; Larry was a generous man who never inquired about her extravagant purchases that were automatically paid for by his secretary. Caroline attended the important social and charity events—always perfectly groomed. Her increasing depression was treated with medication prescribed by a psychiatrist in another town.

Power and Interest Invested in Relationships

Another aspect of relationship power involves the degree of interest and investment in the relationship each of the partners has. Usually the individual who has the least interest holds the greater power (Agnew, 1999). Lesser interest can exist for different reasons. The person may not have formed a strong emotional attachment or may, in general, be emotionally aloof. Having a greater amount of resources in the relationship may also in some cases reduce the interest invested. Yet another reason for lower interest can be found in the desirable alternatives an individual perceives to be available to him or her outside the relationship.

In some instances, a married woman who is in daily contact with a higher-status man—perhaps within a work relationship—may become sexually interested in the man and embark upon an extramarital affair. While she is considering what evolutionary theorists would call "mate-switching," her interest level in the relationship with her husband may be reduced, thereby leaving her temporarily with more power in the marital relationship (Buss, 1999).

More frequently, however, the greater power would be linked to the male partner in the relationship. Young women marrying the man they love and having children, frequently sacrifice their careers to some degree in order to raise their children. Even if they work on a part-time basis, their husbands become the primary breadwinners. The woman's bargaining power decreases with the birth of the first child when she requests more help with household chores. Theoretically, every additional child reduces her bargaining power further. At the same time, the husband may perceive several desirable alternatives in his work environment.

The same sexual interest that led the woman into marriage and motherhood may change its character within the context of fear of abandonment by the more powerful partner in the relationship. As women with young children come to realize, they are hit hardest by divorce; "the middle-class professional mother who has 'done the right, responsible thing' and cut back on her career for the sake of her family quickly discovers that when it comes to divorce, no good deed goes unpunished" (Crittenden, 2001, p. 140).

Considering workable definitions of power in heterosexual relationships, Marie Harvey and her colleagues (Harvey, Beckman, Browner, & Sherman, 2002) concluded that two themes of power emerged: power as control and power as decision-making ability. The researchers asked both men and women to describe what would give them the feeling of being powerful in a relationship. Sorting out the responses, it appeared that women included economic independence, physical attractiveness, the ability to provide sex to their spouses, and feeling loved and secure. For the men, the source of power seemed to rest in being able to have control over one's partner and to give orders to one's partner. This particular study involved couples of Mexican origin, and the findings may not be universally applicable, but similarities can be found in some traditional non-Mexican marriage models.

Power and Desire in Sexual Fantasies

Most people engage in sexual fantasies at least at some points in their lives, and as they are functional aspects of sexual desire, professionals have been intrigued about the connection of sexual fantasies and sexual attitudes and behaviors in real life. To gain a greater understanding of the roles of dominance and submission in both men's and women's fantasies, two researchers from the University of California explored the content of sexual fantasies of power—focusing on dominance and submission (Zurbriggen & Yost, 2004).

The participants in the study were 85 men and 77 women between the ages of 21 and 45 who were recruited through advertising to answer open-ended sexual-fantasy questions. As the investigators analyzed the results, they found that men, more so than women, endorsed stereotypical and false beliefs about rape. Men also tended to believe that the sexes are hostile toward one another and held traditional views regarding the women's place in society.

With regard to sexual fantasies, men's fantasies were more sexually explicit than those of women. In addition, there was a gender difference along the dominance-submission continuum. These findings confirm earlier explorations regarding male-female similarities and differences in sexual fantasy (Leitenberg & Henning, 1995).

Men in their fantasies saw themselves much more as dominant and in control than did the women. Women who fantasized about being sexually dominant, interestingly, seemed to focus mainly on their partner's sexual pleasure rather than on their own. This would raise the following question: if women's main goal was men's pleasure rather than their own, how did they explain this as interpretation of their own sexual dominance? Intriguingly, this finding seems to coincide with Jenny's description of her actual sexual experiences, as discussed in Chapter 3, and that of Marian, mentioned earlier.

On the other hand, a woman's fantasizing about her submission to the sexual dominance of a partner does not necessarily mean that in reality it is always the woman's wish to be dominated. There may be other factors in the personal background of the woman that lead her to engage in this particular fantasy without wanting to experience this scenario in reality, as can be seen in the case of Irene, whose experiences were discussed in connection with a girl's formation of her sexual identity (Chapter 4).

Exploring the results regarding desire and pleasure in sexual fantasies, it was found that men described the sexual desire and pleasure of their partners as well as their own. Women, on the other hand, seemed to focus on their own desire and pleasure, not their partners. On the surface, this conclusion seems to contradict the earlier one regarding sexual dominance in women's fantasies. The investigators interpreted this finding to mean that women allowed themselves in fantasy what they could not afford to do in reality, perhaps based on Vance's (1989) argument that it can be dangerous for women to express sexual desire and seek pleasure (Chapter 4).

Unions Made in Heaven?

Some couples appear to have been drawn together by a giant magnet. Their personality characteristics occupy opposite poles on a continuum, which would make it seem that a mixture of the two would reflect a healthy adjustment. The problem is that they usually don't mix well, and each partner tends to remain more or less fixed at his or her end of the continuum.

For a while they might believe that they complement one another well with their differences, as the saying goes, "opposites attract." In relationships with equal power constellations within the couple the situation may evolve along one of two paths. The partners may never agree on anything and argue continuously with eventual eruption and dissolution, or they may take turns in their decision-making activities and this situation might remain workable.

A different path may evolve in relationships where the power is unbalanced. After an initial period of relief from responsibilities, the follower may get tired of always relinquishing control to the leader.

Verna and Marvin: The Compulsive-Impulsive Couple

Verna, a well-educated young professional, had difficulty making decisions. Determined to come up with the perfect solution to every decision-requiring situation that came her way, Verna experienced a tremendous amount of frustration and anxiety. For hours—even days—she would go back and forth, back and forth in her mind over any detail inherent in the situation that might turn a seemingly perfect solution into an egregious error. Her worrying and anxiety became overwhelming, and her physician, diagnosing her with obsessive-compulsive disorder, prescribed medication for her.

Although the medication reduced the level of anxiety somewhat, Verna still was afraid of making decisions. When she met Marvin, Verna thought she had found her missing half. Marvin, a young account executive, seemed so self-assured. Decisions did not appear to bother him in the least; in fact, he arrived at solutions in record time. Verna was duly impressed and when—after a short dating period—Marvin proposed marriage, Verna believed herself to be in decision-making heaven: Never again would she have to worry about it. Her love for Marvin may have been a combination of admiration for him as a person and the freedom from anxiety life with him seemed to promise.

Not surprisingly, Marvin decided on the wedding date, the guest list, and the location for their honeymoon as well as their place of residence. Marvin was successful in his job, and the early promotions he received allowed the couple financially to start planning their family. They agreed on having four children, two boys and two girls. In order to prepare for pregnancy Verna not only gave up her job but also the medication she had been taking. In a short time Marvin found the "perfect" house for them so the move could be accomplished during the early months of Verna's first pregnancy.

Without the medication, Verna's anxiety returned full force. Even if Marvin made all the big decisions for them, she had plenty of opportunity to worry about little decisions, such as food intake, exercise, exposure to environmental toxins, etc., that might negatively affect the pregnancy or the developing fetus. At about the same time she discovered little things she did not like about their house. When she voiced her opinion to Marvin, he responded with statements that the house was the best solution at the time and they would probably sell it and move into another one in the next couple of years. Marvin assured Verna that she was not really knowledgeable about property values.

During the time when they were dating and the years of their early marriage their sex life had been great. Marvin had a strong sex drive, and Verna, feeling relieved of her anxiety about making decisions, felt adventurous sexually as well as flattered by Marvin's frequent sexual overtures. Lately, however, her worries seemed to have taken the luster off her earlier excitement. Without the medication, her anxiety made it difficult for her to relax, and she worried about her newborn son in the next room.

With her second and third pregnancies, her anxiety steadily increased. Verna had to make many small decisions during the day. If one of the children had a cough, should she call the pediatrician? How long should she wait for the cough to subside before calling? In her frustration, she often called Marvin at work. He was not pleased and scolded her for her uncertainties. The children became sensitive to Verna's worries about health issues and complained about little aches and pains more frequently. Verna's confidence in her own ability to cope with their daily life took a nosedive. Verna and Marvin decided not to have a fourth child after all.

As the level of her daily frustrations about the children's well-being increased, she noticed that Marvin had been in the habit of making major purchases without requesting her input. In the spring, citing concerns for the children's health and safety, Marvin had initiated negotiations with contractors for an in-ground swimming pool in their backyard. With their own swimming pool, he explained, they would not have to worry about any germs the kids were likely to pick up in a public pool.

What most surprised Verna about these decisions was the speed with which they were arrived at and executed. Just about 2 months earlier Marvin had come home with a big, brand-new vehicle instead of the car he had been driving for the past couple of years. He explained that, in view of Verna's concerns with the children's health, they needed a safe, reliable means of transportation. Verna asked him why, if that had been his concern, did he not trade *her* car in for a new, safer automobile. Marvin countered that in an emergency she would probably not be able to drive and would call him at work—he would be the one to drive them where they needed to go.

A couple of weeks after that Marvin called to instruct her to stay home for the rest of the day and make room in their basement for the delivery of some exercise equipment he had ordered. Verna wondered about the cost of all these things and if Marvin perhaps was a bit too impulsive in his spending. Furthermore, the exercise equipment required more space than she had expected. There would not be much space for the children to play in the basement on rainy days.

She expressed her concerns to Marvin when he returned from work. He thought she would understand that buying the exercise equipment was a good investment in their health. Having the equipment at home saved him the time it took to drive back and forth to a gym. Besides, Marvin added, Verna could do with some physical exercise to perk her up; lately she seemed lethargic when it came to sex.

Although Verna had been a capable and respected young professional who had handled her own finances prior to marrying Marvin, now she had absolutely no knowledge about their financial standing. She did not know what savings or investments they had, if they had any debts, and if so how much. She was uninformed about her husband's salary. She did not even know how much their monthly mortgage payments were. Marvin handled all of that.

Verna wondered if she needed to be concerned about this. Where she had once been grateful for not having to make significant decisions, she now felt that Marvin might be too impulsive with his decisions. In addition, she did not like the way he was patronizing her lately and acting as if she was too incompetent to even be considered in decisions about the family's purchases and finances.

Verna's shrinking self-esteem and her resentment toward Marvin made for poor bedfellows. Her feelings for him cooled and any sexual interest that may still have been there vanished. Verna focused on how Marvin had taken advantage of her anxiety and decision-making difficulties. She did not fully comprehend that by not working on overcoming her anxiety and learning to make decisions rationally and realistically, she had willingly abdicated her power in exchange for the relief of her frustrations. Her insecurity and dependence on Marvin had cost her the self-esteem she once had as well as the feelings she once had for her husband.

It is not surprising that Verna handed the decision-making aspect of their marriage over to Marvin. Even if she had not been so obsessive about her own fears of making the wrong decisions, in our culture men are generally seen as the decision-makers. And those who are capable of seemingly knowing quickly what to do in various situations are admired in business and industry. As one male account executive stated, "You are expected to make decisions quickly to inspire trust in those around you. It does not matter as much that you make the best possible decision as it matters that you respond adroitly. If your choice was not the perfect one, you have time later to adjust the details so it will appear to be the most efficient one."

The Controlling Force of Obsessive Love

A type of relationship that is based on unbalanced power can be one where possessive love is one of the main ingredients of the relationship. At first glance, one might assume that the jealous partner would be the powerless one in the relationship because of that person's need for the other. However, through experience the jealous partner has had plenty of practice converting the need into expressed demands that give the appearance of control.

The jealous individual needs little provocation in order to demand proof constantly that his or her suspicions are groundless without ever really accepting anything as proof, short of having the desired object or person in his or her constant possession. In order to feel secure, having absolute control over the possession is necessary. If the target possession is a person, the goal is to have that person under constant observation or confined to a place from which escape is impossible.

At the beginning it is easy for the target person to mistake the jealous individual's intense attention for sincere love and devotion. In fact, the intensity may resemble a passion deep enough to engulf and sweep up the target person along with the jealous individual into one great, fervent romance. Secretly, so many of us are longing for that passionate love that will lift our experiences high above what "ordinary" loving couples feel. Novels and movies never tire of portraying couples in ecstatic embraces, indicating passionate romance. Having paid the price of admittance, shouldn't the movie fan be entitled to some of those experiences too? As one client phrased it, "I want an enduring passionate intimate relationship—is that asking too much for from life?"

What makes the attention appear so ardent and so seductive is really a passionate obsession the jealous person has with him- or herself. Viewed as a possession, the target person becomes part of the jealous individual, and the love affair is not so much a loving relationship between two individuals as it is an expression of extended self-love on the part of the jealous person. The "possession" is held onto as a means for need fulfillment and an opportunity for self-aggrandizement.

What differentiates possessive love from healthy love is a missing ingredient—trust. A person consumed by obsessive love knows no trust. There is a strong belief in the jealous person that he or she not only needs but is entitled to the love and attention of the target person. There may also be a belief that it would be best for the target person to comply with these needs; but trust is not a part of it. Thus, for the controller to achieve what seems necessary, complete control over the target person is a basic requirement.

Obsessive and jealous male lovers may resort to stronger control measures, including emotional as well as—at times—physical restraining measures over their target persons. The only thing worse than being in a relationship with a jealous controller is being involved with a jealous controller who has already been disappointed. Every perceived "betrayal" increases the need for control, and the target person becomes the one who is made to pay for previous rejections.

Jeff and Libby and the Punching Bag

Jeff and Libby were engaged and would soon be married. Libby was a warm, caring, and fun-loving young woman. She was always ready to help when her friends were in need, and she pitched in at work to help her coworkers meet deadlines. On the surface, people judged her to be a "carefree spirit," but underneath she was a serious person, concerned about others and about the environment. Jeff had been married before; he did not talk much about it. He appeared sincere, quiet, and protective; one could trust his word, Libby thought. She was strongly attracted to Jeff, who proved to be an ardent lover. His personality structure did include a touch of perfectionism, though.

During a visit to Jeff's apartment Libby noticed a punching bag. "What is this for?" she asked. In answering, Jeff told her a little more about his previous marriage. His ex-wife had been unfaithful. One day she made him so angry that he punched a hole in the bathroom door. They had been involved in an argument about her affair when she locked herself in the bathroom. Jeff was so frustrated and upset; he felt he had to hit something to release his anger: "Better the door than a human being," he reasoned. It sounded like tremendous restraint, a great act of self-discipline. He had controlled his feelings insofar as he was able to find a more appropriate target. "What strength!" Libby thought when he told her the story.

Once they were married, they established their routines. Libby learned that Jeff did not take easily to change and did not want her to venture out alone. His job was stressful, and the routines gave him a sense of relief. Because some contact with his ex-wife was necessary for their children's sake, Jeff made it his responsibility to answer all phone calls. Often after a phone call from his ex-wife Jeff disappeared into the room with the punching bag. Over time Libby learned to recognize some of the stress signs. She felt good that Jeff's visits with the punching bag were not triggered by any of their interactions.

Jeff's habit of answering the phone at home prompted Libby to keep up with most of her communications with friends during her lunch break at work. She felt the time in the evenings belonged to Jeff and her with as few interruptions as possible. Recently, a male cousin had moved to town. He had called Libby at home, requesting some information about his new environment. A few times on the weekend Libby had gone with him to show him different places for shopping or to point out different agencies that could be helpful to him. Jeff had been displeased about the attention she had given her cousin, and she tried to keep it to a minimum. The weekends were Jeff and Libby's special time.

A few times Libby met with her cousin during her lunch breaks to help him get oriented. One day Jeff had dropped in at her place of work unexpectedly and observed Libby and the cousin sitting outside chatting and laughing. Jeff was not pleased. Later at home he accused Libby of caring more for her cousin than for their marriage. That evening was the first time Jeff went to the punching bag without a reason from his ex-wife. When Libby heard the sounds of the punches she knew it was in response to her interaction with her cousin. Later Jeff initiated sex. Libby complied, although she was not really in the mood for it.

Little by little, Libby's feelings for Jeff changed. The sounds of the punching bag that night had given rise to anxiety, which overshadowed the openness and depth of her feelings for Jeff. The level of her sexual interest decreased gradually due to the tension she felt. As her participation in their lovemaking became less enthusiastic, Jeff became more confrontational in his accusations. It was only a matter of time until she heard the sound of the punching bag again in response to one of their interactions. She grew tense but did not confide in anyone about her anxiety and the reason for it. She made mistakes at work that were uncharacteristic of her.

One evening Libby stayed at her job longer than usual, trying to catch up with a backlog of work. When she arrived home she found Jeff waiting at the door. He pulled her inside and accused her of having an affair with her cousin. He was quite certain of it; her behavior was very similar to his ex-wife's behavior at the time that she had betrayed Jeff. Libby tried to defend herself without success.

That evening Jeff did not make it to the punching bag. The next morning Libby arrived at work trying to conceal a black eye and a bruised nose. She was sent to the company physician, who diagnosed and taped a few broken ribs in addition to treating her facial bruises. He wrote in his report that her injuries were most likely the result of domestic violence. The nurse gave Libby the phone number of a shelter for battered women. Libby was embarrassed, ashamed, insulted—what was she to do? Should she press charges and divorce Jeff? Should she admit that she made mistakes and therefore should give Jeff another chance? Should she become a willing participant in her own victimization?

Remembering Rutter's (1989) statement mentioned earlier in this chapter about the possible consequences when women's deference to men becomes internalized as a cultural value, we can appreciate the temptation experienced by Verna, Caroline, Megan, and Libby to be drawn into relationships of unbalanced power and become victimized emotionally or physically or both by their controlling partners. It is also noteworthy that some of the women—namely, Megan, Libby, and Lenore (introduced in Chapter 4)—had married divorced men without obtaining much detailed information about the reasons for their husbands' previous divorces. Are women perhaps too ready to believe that the earlier break-up had to be the other woman's—the ex-wife's—fault?

At the beginning of their relationships the women experienced a healthy interest in sex, and their admiration for the strong or powerful partner was a part of it. But over time their interest eroded due to the loss of their independence and personal significance, which they allowed to be taken away from them. In most of these cases the controlling men had managed slowly and subtly to isolate the women socially from coworkers, friends, and even relatives, thus stripping them of available and much needed support.

Some women after having experienced painful and disappointing relationships may be able to redevelop their initial healthy sexual desire. Others may perceive themselves as having been led astray once by sexual desire and may not only extinguish their desire for a particular man but may decide not to ever experience it again in the future with any man because their own desire had betrayed them. Experiences of reduced sexual desire that once were person or situation specific may become generalized to include any sexual contact with any male partner. Burnt by it once, these women might consider sexual desire to be something too dangerous to play with again.

7
Intra-Personal Considerations Relevant to Sex Therapy

As outlined in previous chapters, social and cultural factors exert a significant influence on women's sexuality. Added to this influence is a host of personal considerations and personality characteristics that come into play in ways that are unique to each woman and affect each woman in a different manner. Thus, each woman becomes a unique mixture of social, cultural, and personal influences. Furthermore, as time passes, this unique mixture that constitutes a woman changes physically, mentally, and emotionally, so that today's woman may hardly resemble yesterday's girl.

Personality Characteristics Affecting Sexual Attitudes and Behavior

The word *personality* has been used in many different ways and contexts. Its meaning can range from descriptions of one's charm or charisma to constellations of characteristics that define one person as unique and different from all others. How does a person's personality develop? How do the contributing factors combine in such unique ways for various individuals? Most theorists would agree with the statement that "the outcome is determined by the experiential history of the person, the kind and degree and pattern of experiences she has had, impinging upon and affecting the development and maturation of the basic or innate qualities that were there at birth" (Williams, 1983, p. 22).

All the more surprising is it that little has been said and written about the relationship between personality style and sexual difficulties. As an exception, some studies have revealed a linkage between specific sexual dysfunctions and discernible characteristic symptom profiles (Derogatis, 1981). For instance, men diagnosed with inhibited sexual excitement also showed high phobic anxiety and somatization and low hostility, whereas men complaining of premature ejaculation showed the opposite pattern with low phobic anxiety but high levels of hostility. Similarly, women diagnosed with inhibited orgasm showed high levels of depression and interpersonal sensitivity.

The connection between certain kinds of psychological stress and sexual discomfort is not a causal one but is an indication that certain personality characteristics may be consistent with particular sexual complaints. When there is a sexual problem, it usually is consistent with the individual's particular personality style and should be considered in the context of that person's overall character structure. "This is particularly important when determining therapeutic interventions, because these should be applicable not only to the sexual symptom itself, but also to the person's overall psychological functioning" (Kuriansky, 1988, p. 25).

Individuals' personality characteristics influence what type of partner they choose. Couples pick one another to fulfill not only their mental and emotional needs but also their sexual needs. An obsessive person carries his or her general rigidity into lovemaking routines; if he or she has chosen a more spontaneous partner to complement his or her own style, their sexual interaction may well be troubled by the expressions of their individual personality characteristics.

Women, who want to merge completely with their partners, and perhaps combine this desire with a fear of abandonment, may choose to engage in self-sacrificing behaviors toward their partners and fail to develop their own identity. Women with histrionic personality characteristics may experience an exaggerated need for love and attention, similar to an addiction to drugs or alcohol. Life becomes intolerable without the fix—a lover verbalizing undying love—to the point that the women experience withdrawal symptoms including depression (Kuriansky, 1988).

As another reminder about the complexity inherent in the lives of so many women, Jenny, the young woman introduced in Chapter 3, may partly fit this scenario.

From Penis Envy to Jealousy, Narcissism, and Shame

Discussions about personality invariably go back to the influences of Sigmund Freud. In his theories on psychosexual development, Freud (1963) made the connection between certain neuroses in women and feelings of biologic inferiority and penis envy. Even when the woman does not consciously envy the man's penis, a remnant of that envy remains with her in the form of jealousy, Freud reasoned. The character trait of jealousy was considered to be much more prevalent in the mental make-up of women than in that of men.

Thus, in the early psychological considerations of female development, women bore the external symbol of their own inferiority—the missing penis—and were endowed instead with the unflattering character trait of jealousy resulting from the lack of the penis. According to Freud, other character traits resulting from women's penis envy were narcissism, a preoccupation with the self and the strong need to be loved, vanity—expressed in the value women put on their physical attractiveness—and shame, which had as its purpose the camouflage of the women's genital deficiency.

Although Freudian theory drew much criticism, some aspects of it seem to remain with us today. In Greek mythology, Narcissus was a male youth who fell in love with his own reflection, but his gender did not prevent that the personality traits of narcissism, passivity, and masochism became central elements in Helene Deutsch's theory of femininity. Deutsch worked with Freud in Vienna and was strongly influenced by Freud's ideas. Deutsch saw women's sexuality as culminating in orgasms, which were part of the natural consequences of sexual activity—pregnancy and childbirth. For men, the sexual act was an end in itself but women's orgasms—although pleasurable—were more like a vicarious reflection of the man's orgasm in nature (Sayers, 1991).

It is not the intent here to provide an extensive history of psychological considerations regarding women's sexuality. However, it is of interest to consider the links between female sexuality and character variables conceived of and explained by the thinkers of earlier times, who interestingly did not appear to assume similar links to be relevant to male sexuality. The consideration of personality characteristics and their effects in general—whether we look at males or females—is certainly relevant to the work of sex therapists today.

Julie: Obsessive-Compulsiveness Extinguishing Sexual Desire

Julie, having come from a chaotic, alcoholic family background, had adopted the principles of control and orderliness as her guidelines for life. Being in control of the situations in her life provided the safety and security she had craved as a child. Order was necessary to maintain control. Her daily activities were scheduled and organized for maximum efficiency. Her day was not over without the dinner dishes being cleaned and put away and the family's clothes for the next day laid out ready to be worn. Although she loved her husband, she was not able or willing to interrupt her routines for sexual intercourse; sex had to wait until the end of the day when everything else was taken care of.

Having given birth to three children, Julie did not consider sexual intercourse a top priority, but remaining in control was. Her need for control did not allow her to delegate chores to others because they were either not completed to her satisfaction or they did not get done on time. Julie's thoughts and behaviors reflected obsessive-compulsive personality traits. In her profession as a nurse, those traits came in handy, but in her family life, and especially her sexual life, they became troublesome.

Julie's husband felt that he was the least important aspect of her life. To ease Julie's load, he offered to help with chores, but his help was not satisfactory. Often he would go to bed hoping that Julie would join him early enough for sex. At times he had fallen asleep by the time she retired to the bedroom; at other times she complied with his wishes for sex, but it was obvious that she was exhausted. He suggested marriage counseling and Julie was offended at his suggestion. She believed that she did everything she could think of for the family, except set aside quality time for lovemaking with her husband.

On the rare occasions when Julie and her husband were able to go off on a weekend alone the couple's sex life improved. This is a situation frequently encountered in other sexually troubled couples. But as Julie's husband stated when he started divorce proceedings, a marriage cannot live on vacations alone. Julie did not want a divorce. She wanted to keep the children's father in the house with them. But it was too late. Julie's obsessive-compulsive traits and the low priority level assigned to sex proved to be a losing combination. Counseling, as her husband had suggested, or sex therapy without attention to the deeper issues would probably not have been successful.

Personality Traits and Exchange Theory

Narcissism, another female personality trait proposed by Freud, might play a role in female sexual excitement, as it is also related to aspects of exchange theory mentioned in Chapter 3. For example, a woman who is aware and appreciative of her physical attractiveness may spend much time and energy in maintaining and enhancing it because her beauty is an asset in the marriage market. Taking care of a bargaining asset such as one's physical beauty can assume narcissistic proportions, and the seductive power over a male that it affords can prove to be a sexual turn-on for the woman. Anita, one of the members in a women's support group mentioned in Chapters 6 and 10, found the arousal power of her physical beauty sexually stimulating.

As an application of an economic perspective, exchange theory has been adapted to social relationships. The basic premise of exchange theory is that people will use their resources and assets to bargain for rewards and advantages in their relationships. The exchange transactions of costs and rewards are seen as forming the basis and stabilizing factors in a relationship (Becker, 1991; Sabatelli & Shehan, 1993). In cases where one person feels that the exchange balance is one-sided, the relationship is likely to be unhappy and will eventually dissolve. Thus, whether a dissatisfied couple divorces can be analyzed in exchange theory terms (Brehm, Miller, Perlman, & Campbell, 2002).

Self-Concept and Sexuality

What makes up a woman's sexual concept of herself? In our culture, women's concern with the weight and shape of their bodies and their physical attractiveness is well accepted and exploited by commercial enterprises. Most individuals turn their focus on external features. Usually, questions about a woman's skills as a lover or companion are secondary to these external physical concerns.

A person's self-concept has an impact on that person's behaviors, relationships, and sexuality. A woman who feels comfortable with her body and believes she is entitled to sexual pleasure will take an active role in attaining sexual fulfillment. As a result, she is likely to have a more satisfying sexual relationship than a woman who lacks those positive feelings about herself. Women who during sexual activities are concerned about displaying their bodies from the most advantageous point of view and hiding physical flaws become spectators rather than participants in sexual play. While engaged in observing, they miss out on the pleasures to be experienced as a participant (Trapnell, Meston, & Gorzalka, 1997). Not surprisingly, research has demonstrated that self-esteem and self-confidence are correlated with higher sexual satisfaction and absence of sexual problems.

Perceived Age-Related Decline in Attractiveness and Reduced Sexual Interest

As women observe and evaluate their own physical appearance, concerns about their body esteem, or body image, focus on several components: weight concerns, sexual attractiveness, and physical condition. With increasing age, these concerns also increase; and in Western society women who approach midlife are confronted with the double jeopardy of ageism and sexism, causing their physical self-esteem to plummet.

How strongly the age issue is related to perceived physical attractiveness and in turn to sexual desire was demonstrated in a longitudinal study involving 307 heterosexual middle-aged women (Koch, Mansfield, Thurau, & Carey, 2005). Regardless of their particular age, women who thought they were less attractive now than they had been 10 years earlier also indicated a decline in sexual desire or frequency of sexual activity. Women who perceived themselves as attractive were more likely to experience an increase in sexual desire and frequency of sexual activity. Perceived physical attractiveness did not change significantly based on the woman's menopausal status, according to the investigators.

Shame-Proneness and Sexual Desire

Although links between gender role stress and shame-proneness have been found to exist in both men and women, for women shame-proneness was most strongly related to difficulties in living up to female gender role norms, especially with regard to physical attractiveness (Efthim, Kenny, & Mahalik, 2001).

Women's responsibilities of taking care of a home and family, often in addition to outside employment, leave little time and energy for the physical exercise necessary to maintain the slender and fit bodies of their youth. Moreover, the physical exhaustion women experience at the end of the day often leads to overeating out of tiredness. Memories of their reflections in the mirror accompany the women to bed and suppress any notion of carefree participation in sexual activities. In such a frame of mind, who would want to display a less than perfect body for the sake of an activity that does not create a significant product as it did in the child-bearing years of their marriage? The combination of negative feelings with self-consciousness and today's hectic lifestyles makes sex a low priority for many women.

Women's negative thoughts connected with sexual activities form part of the cognitive component in what John Bancroft (2002), the former director of the Kinsey Institute, called the "psychosomatic circle" leading to inhibition of sexual responses. Many women's beliefs about themselves and their own attractiveness as they are expressed in their cognitive processes lead to feelings of depression and anxiety, ultimately impacting their moods and attitudes about sex negatively.

Furthermore, women's negative thoughts are facilitated by the media, as the media shapes our perceptions of female attractiveness and desirability with a focus on weight. In the early 1980s, the body weight of the average model was 8% less than that of the average American woman. Now the average model weighs 23% less than the average woman. Famous full-figured actresses of the past, such as Marilyn Monroe, Elizabeth Taylor, and Sophia Loren, have been replaced by today's ultra-thin actresses.

Women Relinquishing Their Sexual Desire Through Silence

For most women sex is much more than the question of whether or not she is in a sexual relationship or whether or not she is experiencing orgasms. Mental and emotional aspects of her life contribute positive or negative factors that affect her sexual moods. For a woman, it is not as easy as it is for men to compartmentalize sex into its appropriate time and place. As with men, though, for women sex is linked to their sense of self-esteem. But where for men performance anxiety may become an issue, women—as described above—are self-conscious primarily about their attractiveness and secondarily about their skillfulness.

In addition, women feel obligated to please or satisfy a man for fear of being abandoned, as we saw with Beth, the young woman whose story is described in an earlier section of the book that examines women with high sexual desire (Chapter 3). That same fear may also keep them from expressing their wishes for more enjoyable sexual activities than those provided by their partners. Fear also prevents the development of true emotional intimacy, and a lack of communication about what is pleasurable widens the gap between partners. Not asking for what is enjoyable is the best guarantee for not getting it. Women's silence about their wishes is just the first step on the road to relinquishing their sexual desire.

Hannah: Not Worthy To Ask for More

Hannah had enjoyed sex in the early part of her marriage to Burt; they spent evenings and weekends pleasing each other sexually. This was before he became CEO of the company he worked for. His new position demanded increased time investments. After having ascended so far on the career ladder, Burt did not want to leave anything to chance. His energy was continually spent in efforts to cement his power and control in the organization. During his long hours at the office, Hannah kept busy at home with their two children. Sex became less of an opportunity to explore and enjoy each other's bodies than a means to relieve Burt's tension.

Their emotional closeness deteriorated under the pressure of time and they were not prepared for the tragedy that struck. While on an errand one day, Hannah was involved in a motor vehicle accident; the driver of another car had run a red light. Their young son, who was in the car with Hannah, was killed instantly. Hannah sustained severe injuries and underwent several surgeries which left her with scars on her face and body. Not surprisingly, Hannah and Roger's sex life was further affected by depression over the tragedy. Roger's depression lifted over time as he applied himself even more to his work. Although she was not at fault, Hannah blamed herself for her son's death. The combination of her guilt feelings, the loss of her child, and the loss of her attractiveness severely impacted her self-esteem. She felt she was not worth much attention from Roger, and although she made herself available for sexual intercourse, her desire decreased more and more as Roger's brief sexual routine left her unfulfilled. She denied herself the right to ask for more.

Establishing a False Sense of Security by Searching for Partner's Faults

Other individuals with low self-esteem reason that if they detect some imperfections in their partner, it will give them greater security: a partner who is less than perfect may be less likely to leave because it would be difficult to find another accepting mate. Of course, it is not sufficient that one partner sees the imperfections of the other. To maintain this false sense of security, the mate must be made aware that he or she indeed possesses these imperfections.

Mary: Looking for Imperfections

When Mary first met Joe she could not believe that somebody so wonderful would be interested in her. Joe was the hero who would rescue her from her fears of not measuring up. Joe, however, had his own insecurities, which he tried to hide from Mary. For a while they seemed to have found paradise; they moved in together and their sex life was terrific.

Mary was probably the first to experience a reappearance of her old doubts. She became moody; some of Joe's habits irritated her. She reasoned that it was best to tell him about the habits that disturbed her, as she explained, "I would like to know when I do something that irritates Joe so I can stop doing it." Joe did not respond in the expected manner; he thought she was nagging him. He defended himself by pointing out some of Mary's habits that he considered to be less than delightful. Joe's response shocked her. Mixed in with the fear of losing him was anger about his insensitivity. Here she was trying to help him get rid of his irritating habits only to be confronted with her own shortcomings.

Mary maintained her watchfulness. As one would expect, their arguments increased in frequency. Another consequence of Mary's vigilance regarding Joe's irritating habits was that her own feelings for him seemed to grow less passionate. She found it difficult to feel sexual desire for someone whose faults she focused on so intently. Joe, on the other hand, felt discouraged as well as betrayed. Sweet Mary, who seemed to adore him in the beginning, now had nothing but criticism for him. He knew that he was not Prince Charming, but he did not need constant reminders of this. He decided to move out. Their living-together relationship that had started out so promising had lasted less than 2 years.

The insecurity that each of them felt inside did not make them strong together, as they might have hoped. Instead they used it to tear each other down and to destroy the love they once had for each other. In their struggle for security they opted for the insecurity of competition.

Partner Choice and Its Impact on Sexuality

In the absence of professional matchmakers found in some other societies, individuals in Western societies enter the marriage market with their own blueprint of a suitable partner in hand. For some the search has proven to be more difficult than expected; and to alleviate these difficulties, newer versions of the traditional matchmaker have appeared to serve the public.

Characteristics such as social class, age, physical attractiveness, and education are bargaining factors in the marriage market. In the marital exchange, traditionally linked to gender, women historically have traded their ability to bear children and perform domestic duties, along with physical attractiveness and sexual accessibility, for protection and economic support.

There are, however, gender-related disadvantages in the traditional exchange. While men can take time to look around for a partner because their occupational *potential* can translate into marital security; women, on the other hand, are working against time, as it reduces the traditional female assets of attractiveness and childbearing capacity, which decrease in value as the woman ages.

When considering a man as a potential future husband, the criteria women apply may be different from the ones they use when choosing a lover. The process of lover selection is often unconscious. The woman becomes attracted to certain personality characteristics and behaviors demonstrated by the man, and often it may be the man's ardent pursuit or—in some other cases—the challenge of his lack of attention that makes him so desirable. Passion is the facilitator of the affair-type relationship, whereas stability of character, similar lifestyle expectations, and overall reliability are the preferred ingredients for a husband. And although a woman might have deep loving feelings for her future husband, her sexual attraction and desire for him might be of a calmer variety than what she would feel for a lover.

"Sensible" Choices and Sexual Desire

Although the impact of mate selection on a woman's sexual interest has been discussed in other parts of this book, it deserves our focus here, as it illustrates how the developing emotions within the relationship with the selected partner set the stage for the dynamics that are at work in desire-phase situations.

At times, a woman may make what she considers to be a "sensible" decision about a future husband. When motherhood becomes a deciding factor in mate selection, attention is given to characteristics such as stability of income and character, health, family background, and similar considerations. Physical attractiveness and passion—deciding factors in love affairs—may play a secondary role. Additionally, passionate love affairs may have brought disappointment and despair at the breakup point. Some women don't want to repeat that painful experience and may instead make more sensible choices in selecting a husband and father of their children.

One element that at times works against these carefully laid plans is that the kind of blind love that is often part of infatuation and that works as a buffer by masking undesirable traits and habits in the other—at least, for a while—is absent from the well-planned marriages. Therefore, disenchantment may set in earlier here than in other passion-regulated unions.

Lynn: Resentment

Lynn was not sexually inexperienced; she had been married before and after her divorce had been involved in several romantic relationships. At the beginning of a new relationship Lynn's sexual desire seemed normal, but her excitement faded as time went on. It did not bother her to end relationships; she knew how to pleasure herself to orgasm and she found meaning and satisfaction in her career.

However, in her middle thirties, she was painfully aware that her "biological clock" was ticking, and she did not want to miss out on motherhood. Just in time, she met an eligible man with a promising career of his own. He was divorced and had to pay support for a child from his previous marriage, but he seemed to possess many of the characteristics of a good provider.

Although Lynn was not passionately in love with Robert, she liked his kindness. They shared many of the same values and seemed compatible enough to get married. Robert would have preferred for this marriage to remain childless, but he agreed to become a father again because he considered it unfair to deprive Lynn of the experience of motherhood.

The newness of the relationship combined with the promise of motherhood was sufficient to stimulate Lynn's sexual interest in Robert. There was a period of disappointment when Lynn did not become pregnant right away, but she pursued her goal with increased frequency of sexual intercourse. It paid off; she got pregnant and gave birth to healthy twin boys.

Perhaps due to her increased testosterone level during her pregnancy, her level of sexual desire remained relatively high during this period. She restructured her career so that her home became her work base with occasional visits to the employer's offices. Lynn was happy. Her natural preoccupation with her new babies kept her from noticing Robert's weight loss, tension, and decreased ability to concentrate. By now the end of her thirties was approaching, and Lynn thought it would be good to have another child, a daughter. When she addressed her wishes in conversations with Robert, a self-employed contractor, he admitted that the financial stress of another child was more than he could handle at the time. His condition deteriorated further. With medical help, Robert regained his strength; but it was too late. Lynn's fortieth birthday had passed and her physician advised against another pregnancy.

Lynn became depressed, although she put up a good front for her friends and neighbors. Only with her sons did she feel lively and fulfilled. Robert was well enough to desire sex, but Lynn was in no mood to participate. She put it off as long as she could, eventually giving in from time to time. The periods between sexual intercourse became longer and longer. On those occasions that she decided to go ahead with sex, she discouraged foreplay, which made the whole interaction more strained and less pleasurable.

It did not take long for Robert to realize that he was not desirable to Lynn and that his attempts to initiate sex were a nuisance to her. Of course, he felt hurt and withdrew, approaching her only occasionally and without success. There were periodic angry outbursts when Robert brought up the neglect of his sexual needs; Lynn countered with his insensitivity to her wishes, but nothing changed. Robert suggested counseling and Lynn contacted a therapist. In her sessions she avoided discussion of the sexual issue under the pretext that she wanted to work on other issues first. And there were other issues, mostly anger-related situations with people in her environment. For years she had suppressed her angry feelings under a pleasing façade, too afraid to express them overtly. She admitted to strong feelings of resentment toward Robert because his illness had deprived her of having a daughter.

Of course, she did not dare communicate that resentment openly to her husband, but she also did not change her feelings. Lynn had placed herself in a stalemate position. She could not allow herself to express the real reasons for her anger to Robert for fear that he might leave the marriage. On the other hand, she did not want to relinquish her anger because in her mind it served as justification for her refusal to engage in sex with Robert. After a few more sessions Lynn discontinued treatment. Like Claire, whom we encountered in Chapter 5, Lynn had built up walls of anger between herself and her husband. Every time Lynn saw a pretty little girl she felt deprived of the daughter she wanted, and she blamed Robert because he had not been willing or ready to have another child with her.

Ruth and Edith: Potential for Future Husbands

Ruth and Edith became friends when both their husbands, who worked for the same company, were transferred to a different part of the country. Ruth had married Pete when she found herself pregnant. Pete did not arouse passion in her like some of the other men she had dated, but he was a good man, hardworking and reliable. Although she did not get pregnant while they were dating, Edith had decided to get married to Larry for very similar reasons. She felt it was time to start a family, and Larry—although not a passionate lover—was a caring and trustworthy man. Over the years, Ruth, a passionate woman, had tried to make sexual intercourse with Pete more playful and interesting, but she did not succeed. Pete had certain ideas about sexual behaviors, and he was not willing to deviate from his routine. Edith's sex life with Larry proved equally boring to her.

After their friendship had deepened into a devoted sisterly relationship, the two women compared notes about their sex life. They decided to rent videos to watch with their husbands to make their sexual encounters more exciting. When they came together for coffee and discussion of the videos that they had hoped would be of help, they realized that this approach did not work. They thought of other ways to spice up their sex lives but finally had to admit failure. Edith turned to sexual fantasies involving other men when masturbating or even during intercourse with Larry. However, the difference between her fantasies and reality was too great and she struggled through the entire time of intercourse with Larry. She avoided sex with him as much as she could.

Ruth, on the other hand, tried to repress her sexuality and her wishes for passionate lovemaking; as she said, "I did not want to be reminded of what I was missing." Over time her desire for sexual activity dwindled. She realized that she had lost a valuable and, perhaps the most lively, part of herself; but on a daily basis the cost of continuous unfulfilled longing was too high for her to bear.

Neither Ruth nor Edith had suffered from lack of sexual desire in their younger years when they explored life, but both had grown up in families of divorced parents and stepparents. When it came time to settle down and start a family, their choices in husbands set the stage for a sexually unfulfilled life, which completely drained their capacity to feel sexual desire—at least with their husbands. In selecting their mates, Ruth and Edith had unknowingly settled for *conditional* sex, an arrangement in which one partner controls the sexual activities of both. It does not involve exchanges (as in the case of Joan and Fred—discussed in Chapter 5); sex is on the controlling partner's terms or there is no sex at all. Although this situation is quite common—whenever there is a controlling partner in the equation—most couples do not consciously realize that this pattern exists in their relationship (Hajcak & Garwood, 1987).

The Marriage Gradient

Another factor, the tendency for women to marry "up" with regard to age, education, occupation, status, and earning potential, has traditionally influenced marital choice. According to the U.S. Census Bureau (2000, Table 56), in about 57% of U.S. married couples, the husband is 2 or more years older than his wife, and in only 11% of marriages is the wife older than her husband.

Not only do these factors influence marital choice, they exert a strong impact on women's sexuality. Traditionally, most women do not find it erotic to be pursued by a man of lower status or lower educational achievement than their own. Being accompanied to a social gathering by a man of a lower educational level might prove socially embarrassing for a woman. A relationship with a significantly younger man can be equally embarrassing, as the woman might fear the gossiping remarks of having "robbed the cradle." Feelings of embarrassment are not a good breeding ground for sexual excitement or romantic fantasies; power, on the other hand, can be sexually attractive (as illustrated in the section about Barbara Amiel in Chapter 6).

But as gender roles slowly become more alike in our society, other factors, such as affective, sexual, and companionship characteristics, may be increasingly valued. A woman in a high-income bracket might find a nurturing, although lower-wage-earning, husband attractive (Sprecher & Toro-Morn, 2002).

Andrea: Disregarding the Marriage Gradient

Andrea—attractive, bright, and ambitious—was successful in her work as a pharmaceutical representative for a leading company. She became the training director for newly hired representatives and also functioned in a supervisory capacity in clinical trials. Her bosses were impressed with her capabilities and her salary expressed their appreciation. Ralph, Andrea's husband, a gentle, caring man, worked as a male nurse in a convalescent home. His job was to support and encourage patients who struggled with their impediments. Andrea's work schedule was hectic, and often at the end of the day she gratefully released her tension with the help of Ralph's hands as he gave her a massage.

Ralph's job included working different shifts, but on days when he returned home before Andrea he often set the dinner table, prepared a snack or dinner, and drew a relaxing, aromatic bath for her. He took pleasure in pampering her, and they enjoyed their evenings of lovemaking. Andrea loved the touch of his hands and his sexual ministrations, which were passionate, but also considerate of her wishes and needs.

They had been married for almost 2 years when Ralph noticed a subtle change in Andrea's behavior. She seemed less happy when she came home from work. A tiredness and sense of impatience overshadowed her mood. She also seemed less eager to engage in sexual activities. Ralph's increase in caring behavior did not bring about a return to their previously loving interactions. In fact, it seemed to have a negative effect on Andrea's mood and arguments between them ensued. Their sex life deteriorated in frequency and quality until Ralph suggested marriage counseling. Andrea reluctantly agreed. In their first conjoint session Andrea remained rather quiet, letting Ralph do most of the talking. Following this initial session the therapist scheduled individual sessions for each of the spouses.

During Andrea's individual session she admitted that what once had sexually excited her about her marriage had turned into something like boredom; she had become so used to Ralph's loving behavior that she now took it for granted. She mentioned how embarrassed she was about the lack of respect she felt for Ralph lately. In her work she interacted daily with physicians, administrators, and research scientists in the medical and pharmaceutical fields, and she was ashamed to introduce her husband as a "mere nurse" at social gatherings.

The individual session with Ralph revealed that he had been sensitive to the changes in Andrea's behavior and the likely reasons for those changes. He asked the therapist for help on how to cope with the situation. Because of his hurt feelings, his first impulse was to withdraw and to be less attentive toward Andrea, but he also realized that he would not like that changed behavior in himself. He stated that he wanted to live in a relationship like the one they had started out with. Loving and caring behaviors were important parts of his personality—as he saw it.

Several conjoint meetings followed the two individual sessions until Andrea phased out. She had found herself sexually attracted to a physician; since he was a professional contact, she needed to keep any relationship secret from her employer. Apparently, the man was in the process of divorcing his wife, and Andrea hoped that when the divorce became final he would make a commitment to her. In Andrea's case it seemed that she had only temporarily overcome the tendency to follow the general marriage gradient.

Social scientists point out that although people today marry across small class distinctions, they tend not to do so across large class differences. In other words, people choose partners who resemble themselves in many ways, such as similar education, social class, religious orientation, and other background factors. College graduates tend to marry other college graduates, and those without college degrees tend to choose partners without a college education. Similarly, individuals from the upper-middle-class find their mates within the same social class.

But there are exceptions. Some young females from the protective ranks of upper-middle class find the less polished behaviors of young men from the lower classes exciting and irresistible. One could explain this phenomenon with the old saying "opposites attract." What is unfamiliar becomes exotic and erotic.

Melissa: Opposites Attract

Pretty, petite, dark-haired Melissa made such a choice. Fresh out of high school, poised to enter college, she met Jack, who was working for a construction company. He was good-looking in a rough kind of way. It was summer and his short-sleeved shirts allowed for a display of his muscles. Jack's behavior reflected self-confidence—"cocky" was the word Melissa's father used after meeting him. Jack did not seem devoted to Melissa; he treated her sometimes in an aloof, sometimes in a rough manner. His language bordered on the vulgar. It was Jack's display of self-assuredness and his domineering behavior that made Melissa fall hopelessly in love with him. Instead of getting ready for college, she and Jack eloped to get married. Her parents were furious, but when Melissa became pregnant soon after the wedding, they tried to make the best of the family situation.

Melissa's sexual feelings for Jack were as passionate as she could imagine and he was a great lover—at least for a while. A few years into the marriage Jack displayed some behaviors during their sexual interactions that made her feel uncomfortable. He also demanded that she perform some acts that were against her personal and sexual values. When she did not comply, he called her demeaning names. Melissa came to fear those occasions, and what once had been exciting lovemaking times, she now anticipated with some dread and anxiety. Jack accused Melissa of having an interest in other men because she did not seem to desire intercourse with Jack as much as she had in the past. He made some veiled threats about leaving her. After 30 years of marriage, Melissa sought help at a clinic for sexual dysfunction to find ways for rediscovering her sense of sexual interest.

What had first fascinated Melissa when she met Jack had slowly become something she detested. Jack's rude behavior while it was new seemed interesting, but over a prolonged period of time not only did it become as boring as other long-standing behaviors might be—it became repulsive, and even though she still loved Jack in many ways, her sexual desire for him was greatly reduced.

Of course, one could argue that Melissa was probably approaching menopause and the reduction of her sexual desire may have been linked to that biological fact. While this undoubtedly could have had some impact, her desire had been shrinking over several years, and no matter what other conditions come into play, anxiety over a mate's demands and repulsive behavior are hardly contributing factors to improved desire and increased interest in sexual activities.

Other Factors Influencing Women's Sexuality

Women decide to enter sexual relationships for many different reasons, as described earlier. Any one of those reasons contains the potential for causing difficulties in a woman's sexual life. For example, if the reason for being in a sexually intimate relationship is security—financial, emotional, or otherwise—the woman may feel relaxed and rewarded at first upon reaching her goal, but it may only be a matter of time until fears of losing the achieved goal will shift her focus from what has been pleasurable for her to what is pleasurable to the holder of the security. In her striving to remain secure, she is likely to trade her own pleasure away. In this scenario, seduction can swiftly turn into slavery or into abandonment when her value decreases in the eyes of the holder of the security. These situations are very similar to those discussed in women's relationships to power in Chapter 6.

For the woman whose main purpose in a relationship is nurturing another human being, the temptation is great that she will put her partner's needs and wishes above her own. The better she does her job, the more tired and fatigued she will be when the time for lovemaking comes around. And even then, it is more important that her partner feels cared for than that she reaches her own sexual fulfillment.

If the woman's choice for entering a sexual relationship is based on bolstering her own self-esteem, the cost for the enhanced self-image can be extremely high, because she has to be as good or better a sex partner in every sexual encounter.

While she is figuring out new and exotic ways to entice her partner, the capacity for her own pleasure becomes secondary.

Because our culture strongly emphasizes the importance of orgasmic experiences as sexual goals, a woman's inability to come to orgasm can leave her with doubts about being normal. Not only is she losing out by not achieving this goal, she also may become the target for blame when her partner feels threatened about his manhood due to her lack of orgasm. Often, instead of experiencing pleasure, the woman may resort to faking an orgasm, just to appear "normal" in her partner's eyes.

Many of the reasons mentioned here can be considered needs that some women feel compelled to fulfill for what they may consider to be their own peace of mind or their own physical or emotional well-being. But as sex therapist Gina Ogden (1990) explained, "It is not your needs that impair sexual functioning. It is the manipulative role-playing you engage in, in the mistaken belief that your manipulations will help get these needs met" (p. 24).

The various personal aspects that contribute to women's sexual interest can often be traced back to conditions that affected them in their families of origin. For instance, Julie's obsessive-compulsive traits developed in response to having grown up in a chaotic, alcoholic family. In response to that family background, her need for control in life became excessive.

Ruth and Edith had looked for stable personality characteristics when they decided to marry "good men" because of their experiences within divorcing and remarrying families. Melissa, after the enchantment with the unfamiliar wore off, longed to return to the values and behaviors of her middle-class family of origin. And Rachel became almost paralyzed by the fear that she had married a man similar to her father who had risked the family's financial stability.

For some, considering women's sexual attitudes in connection with background factors and personality characteristics may seem overly involved. Working through all these factors while pursuing changes may appear overwhelming and possibly inefficient. However, not considering sexual interest within the context of personal issues and personality traits may reduce behavioral changes attempted in treatment to the level of exercises without deeper meaning.

A Final Note on Personality

Thoughts about personality development usually focus on genetic factors, parental and environmental influences, as well as culturally gender-based aspects. Theoretical approaches attempting to explain why individuals develop along certain paths have led to the formulation of patterns of personality characteristics and even categories of personality disorders. In general, people accept their personalities as a given: "That's the person I am," they pronounce. Whether a given personality pattern has been bestowed upon them by genetics or by destiny, people rarely challenge this assumption. They hold on to it steadfastly as if their lives depended on it.

But what about those people who do not like their personalities or, more important, whose personality characteristics do not work for them but instead make their lives more difficult and interactions with those around them more problematic? Are they doomed to continue on their thorny path? Does it become a question of birthright (for those who like their personality characteristics) or birth defect (for those who are troubled by them)? Or is there hope for change?

Although a detailed discussion of personality constellations and personality theories is beyond the scope of this book, the question remains. Viewing the question as a challenge, one could start with the expressions of individual personality styles. In their behaviors people express elements of their personalities; underlying attitudes, values, and beliefs determine many of the behaviors and thus become parts of people's personality pattern. Behaviors may become ingrained, automatic ways of expression over time, but before they reach that stage they can be changed. Even at the late stage of automatic responding, behaviors can be modified—it just takes more effort and time. People have options to redefine themselves and to change those aspects of their behaviors and elements of their personalities that do not work for them (Maass, 2002).

The first step in the modification process is to be willing to challenge the seemingly inevitable—one's personality; is it really cast in stone? Once individuals are willing to challenge, the next step is to select the behaviors they would like to use to express themselves, perhaps actions they admire in others. It can become a creative process of redesigning oneself.

History provides examples of people who have recreated parts of their personalities. Reportedly, as a young man, John F. Kennedy was fascinated by the attractiveness and magnetism that movie stars seemed to possess. While visiting Hollywood he was determined to meet and observe such stars as Clark Gable, Gary Cooper and other actors he admired (Riggio, 1987). Using these stars as models for his own behaviors and interactions with others, Kennedy—in his own way—became as charismatic as they appeared to him. Observing the behavior of others and noting desirable or successful consequences of the observed person's behavior can provide valuable roadmaps for those who want to improve their own effectiveness. In the 19th century, Amandine-Aurore-Lucile Dupin, a young Frenchwoman who wanted to be a writer had an editor tell her that she would be better off making babies and not literature. Women writers were regarded as second-rate artists and mainly expected to write for female readers. In response to the editor's rejection of her work, the young woman decided to recreate her public image and play the part of a man. She dressed in men's clothes and smoked cigars, drank, and conversed with men. Her first major novel was published under the pseudonym "George Sand," and George Sand remained her public persona throughout her career.

In the late 20th century, another woman commanded the world's interest through manipulation of the images she presented to the public. In addition to becoming a musical star, Madonna Ciccone became a visual symbol, first inventing and then continuously reinventing herself. Rather than let others define her image for her, Madonna assumed control of her own image, one that has had no boundaries assigned to it. In addition, she apparently realized that any one of her "characters" could grow stale over time, and to keep the public from predicting her behaviors, she dramatically altered and reinvented her public persona more than once.

Of course, it is not the recommendation here that the women represented in this book completely change their personalities and their lifestyles. But personality change does go deeper than a new hairdo. The purpose of mentioning the above examples is to demonstrate that it is possible for people, when they realize that some of their personality traits do not work for them, to exchange those for others that offer more self-enhancing properties.

Consider the case history of Julie, described earlier in this chapter: had she been able to conceive of herself as a person who could get what she wanted—control—in ways that would make it easy and desirable for others to share in the family's responsibilities, she would have had more interest and energy left over for pleasurable activities. Unfortunately, mixed in with the need for control was the notion that she was indispensable; nobody could perform the tasks as well or as promptly as she did. Delegating tasks to others may have seemed to Julie to be a reduction of her control.

On the other hand, a more pleasure-oriented personality constellation would have lightened her burden. Julie's obsessive-compulsive traits in reality interfered with the achievement of what she thought she needed most. She lost control over a significant part of the family, her children's father. Possibly with the help of a therapist, as had been suggested by her husband, Julie could have realized that applying more self-enhancing attitudes and behaviors would reward her with far greater levels of control than she had been exercising.

While this discussion is not meant as a recommendation for personality changes in general, it is an invitation to contemplate possible enhancements in the quality of one's lifestyle by assuming the right to design one's interactions with others to one's own satisfaction.

PART III
Toward Resolution

8
Developments in Sexology and Sex Therapy

Along with the emerging sexual awareness brought about by the sexual revolution, the likelihood of difficulties in sexual functioning became a concern. How can one be truly sexually liberated when one feels insecure or self-conscious about one's sexual performance compared to that of the sexual acrobats depicted in the media? In fact, evidence collected during the mid-1970s indicated that approximately 50% of married couples were having significant difficulties in their sexual functioning (McCarthy, Ryan, & Johnson, 1975).

In other words, as people found it easier to discuss sexual issues openly, they were at the same time "liberated" to acknowledge problems within their sexual lives. In response to this development, the new discipline of sex therapy evolved.

Perhaps the level of seriousness of a problem gets defined by who is complaining about it. In the early years of sex therapy most clients were men who experienced difficulties with their sexual performance, such as achieving or maintaining an erection or not being able to ejaculate during intercourse. Often low sexual desire would accompany these difficulties. After all, who would be interested in starting activities that were ultimately not successful? Failure seldom breeds a desire for engaging in activities that result in more failure. In cases where their wives did not have a high level of sexual desire, the situation for men with sexual-performance issues was not as problematic. With the development of pharmaceutical help, however, many men have had their sexual desire re-awakened; and so their wives' low interest in sexual activities becomes more obvious and leads to complaints.

Students of human sexuality today learn about the early work in sex therapy that laid the groundwork for much of the knowledge we make use of now. Some of the early pioneers remained relatively unknown because their work did not become published until much later. For instance, the physician Celia Mosher, mentioned in Chapter 1, kept records of the study she conducted in the late 19th century, but publication had to wait until their discovery within the Stanford University archives in 1974.

The purpose of this chapter is to focus briefly on efforts in research and treatment that have been instrumental in the initiation of the study of sexology, as we know it today. It is by no means an attempt at a comprehensive historical account. Detailed descriptions of the work of the early pioneers in the field in the United States and abroad can be found elsewhere.

European Beginnings

In the latter half of the 19th century, the Austrian psychiatrist Richard von Krafft-Ebing (1840–1902) published the first medical classification of sexual disorders in 1886, the *Psychopathia sexualis* (Hauser, 1994). Some scholars have recognized Krafft-Ebing's writings as a significant influence on Freud's work on sexuality. Krafft-Ebing, who originally had conceived of sexual behavior within a biological-medical framework, broadened his views and became interested in the differentiation between behavior and imagination or the physical and the psychological aspects of sexuality, emphasizing the psychological attitude behind the observable behavior. In an article on the sexual functioning of women he pointed out that the sexual center in the brain was just as important as the sexual organs of the body.

Even though Krafft-Ebing made the shift in focus to the psychological aspects of human behaviors, with regard to women's social status, his view remained centered on biological aspects. He argued that women should receive different legal treatment in cases of wrongdoing because of the biological difference between men and women. For instance, in cases of marital infidelity, women deserved tougher punishment than men for the same offense because women were monogamous by nature and therefore had only a minimal sensual desire, but men's nature was polygamous. Similarly, in his monograph "Psychosis menstrualis. A clinico-forensic Study" (*Psychosis menstrualis. Eine klinisch-forensische Studie*, 1902), he suggested that special laws should be applied to menstruating women because they are not fully responsible for their actions due to their suffering from a periodic madness.

Like Krafft-Ebing, Sigmund Freud came from a medical background but felt drawn to the role of the "basic scientist" and focused on rigorous observation rather than experimentation (Rychlak, 1973). The basis of Freud's theory was a mind–body dualism, and although he developed into a new kind of physician, a healer, he was mostly fascinated with the question of why sickness came about in the first place. Freud's view of human development encompassed a series of psychosexual stages through which individuals pass from infancy to adulthood. According to Freud, the patient's insight was important in facilitating the healing process.

A contemporary of Krafft-Ebing, Henry Havelock Ellis (1859–1939), became known as a leading figure of British sexology (Hall, 1994). Ellis had intended to study medicine but when he obtained the Licentiate of the Society of Apothecaries, the minimum necessary diploma, he abandoned practice to devote himself to work in sexology. His *Studies in the Psychology of Sex*, published in limited, expensive editions, were difficult to obtain, but a short compendium of it was recommended by the medical press as a textbook in medical schools. Ellis has been credited for elevating sexology to the level of a science in its own right.

Early Sexology in the United States

The American medical establishment initially demonstrated reluctance to deal with issues of sexuality, except for cases associated with vice and crime. Official attitudes were characterized by a prescriptive system of moral and cultural values, sexual and economic roles, religious sanctions, hygienic rules, and idealized behavioral patterns called "civilized morality," which was based on a conspiracy of silence and the double standard (Bullough, 1994).

Among the early basic studies of sexual practices in the United States was that of Celia Mosher, mentioned earlier. She had begun her research, which is described in Chapter 1, as a graduate student at the University of Wisconsin in 1892. Another researcher, the obstetrician-gynecologist Robert Latou Dickinson, began his studies in the 1890s, but his statistical data was not published until the early 1930s (Bullough, 1994). Dickinson made the step from research to sex counseling, as he believed that "it was the duty of gynaecologists to do sex counseling in order to preserve marriage, since 'no single cause of mental strain in married women is as widespread as sex fears and maladjustments'" (p. 310). In the early 1920s Dickinson campaigned for better sex education and for birth control.

The physiology of sexual intercourse (later studied by Masters and Johnson) was another area of interest for Dickinson, and using a glass tube in the shape and size of an erect penis to observe the behavior of the vaginal lining and cervix during a woman's orgasm, he was able to prove that female orgasms involved physiological changes in the vagina and the cervix. Together with W. F. Robie and LeMon Clark, Dickinson was instrumental in the introduction of the electrical vibrator. This device produced intense erotic stimulation to the point of orgasm in women who had previously been unable to reach climax. Until the 1920s physicians had treated women who suffered from the common ailment of "hysteria" with manual genital massage to orgasm or what was called then "hysterical paroxysm." With the emergence of the vibrator as a time-saving device, visits to the physician's office could be significantly shortened. Dickinson apparently was willing to entrust women with the instrument.

One of the most widely known researchers of the 20th century, professor of zoology Alfred Kinsey was responsible for collecting the largest database of sexual histories and human sexual behavior, which comprised 17,500 interviews (Reinisch & Beasley, 1990). Results of the extensive survey interviews were published in two volumes: one on male sexuality in 1948 and the other on female sexuality in 1953. Many of Kinsey's data are still relevant today. In his belief that the physical elements of sex could be separated from the others for purposes of study, Kinsey seemed to have anticipated the work of Masters and Johnson.

Masters and Johnson: The Human Sexual Response Cycle

About 45 years ago a clinic for the treatment of human sexual dysfunction was established at Washington University School of Medicine in St. Louis, Missouri. William Masters and Virginia Johnson, well-known pioneers in the field of sex therapy, introduced a novel treatment philosophy: "Although both husband and wife in a sexually dysfunctional marriage are treated, it is the marital relationship that is considered as the patient. Probably this concept is best expressed in the statement that sexual dysfunction is indeed a marital-unit problem, certainly never only a wife's or only a husband's personal concern" (Masters & Johnson, 1970, p. 3).

Based on their findings from years of controlled laboratory experimentation in human sexual physiology, use of dual-sex therapy teams appeared to be the most theoretically effective treatment approach for working with human sexual dysfunction. Thus, husband and wife each had a co-therapist of the same sex as a special interpreter who understood gender-related difficulties in addition to the whole team working with them. During the sessions, one of the co-therapists usually functioned as a silent observer, focusing on some critical points in the verbal interchange that needed further exploration or clarification. Fortified with that information, the silent co-therapist then, in turn, became the active discussant and the previously active co-therapist assumed the observer role.

Included in the treatment philosophy were a time commitment and a certain degree of social isolation required from the participant. The originally prescribed 3-week treatment program was modified to 2 weeks of intense, 7-days-a-week of work. Because about 90% of treated marital units were referred from outside the St. Louis area, participants were isolated from the influences of their regular hometown environments.

In explaining the human sexual response cycle, Masters and Johnson (1966) relied on physiological changes that could be measured and recorded. Their four-phase model covers excitement, plateau, orgasm, and resolution phases. A refractory period is included in the male resolution phase.

Helen Singer Kaplan

The concept of desire as a separate stage was first introduced by Kaplan (1979) as the first stage, the prelude to sexual response, in her three-stage model. Desire did not receive attention as a phase in the Masters and Johnson model. It is important to remember that desire is a prelude and not a necessary first stage, which has to occur before any of the other stages can come into play. Not every sexual response is preceded by desire; one or both partners may agree to engage in sexual activity without experiencing the desire at the moment.

Based on clinical observations, Kaplan (1979) discussed the sexual response cycle in terms of a "biphasic" concept with the notion that excitement and orgasm disorders are actually separate syndromes. Considering the excitement phase and the orgasm phase as separate dysfunctions served to enhance the prognosis of orgasmic disorders in males and females. But from her own work, Kaplan discovered that the prognosis of desire-phase problems is significantly poorer than that of excitement and orgasm-phase disorders. And even in successfully treated cases, the treatment course tended to be more complex and turbulent.

Thus, Kaplan concluded that sexual desire "has a separate physiology, a distinctive pattern of pathogenesis, and special therapeutic requirements" (Kaplan, 1979, p. xviii). Kaplan's conclusions led to a *triphasic model,* encompassing desire, excitement, and orgasm phases.

Fithian and Hartman: Bio-Psycho-Social Approach

At about the same time, another sex therapy team, inspired by the work of Masters and Johnson, developed an intensive, 2-week treatment program. William Hartman and Marilyn Fithian (1974) called their program a "bio-psycho-social approach." As they described their program as a series of steps, activities, and exercises, they explained that because sex is something that people do and not something they talk about, they felt that an action-oriented approach rather than a talk-about-sex approach was indicated.

Many would agree with Fithian and Hartman: people do not talk much about sex while they are in an intimate relationship; indeed, they talk too little about it, leaving plenty of opportunity for misinterpretations of the actions taking place between them. To refrain from talking in such emotionally charged situations may leave the participants with an impression of mystery and uncertainty, conditions difficult to face for some of the inhibited, self-doubting participants with somewhat bruised egos.

Both Masters and Johnson and Hartman and Fithian, in addition to treating couples and individual clients with sexual difficulties, provided training programs for other therapists to become knowledgeable and efficient in their approaches. For two to three decades people could find treatment centers based on the Masters and Johnson/Hartman and Fithian models in several locations throughout the United States and in some foreign countries. It is interesting—and perhaps important—to note that neither the Masters and Johnson book on human sexual inadequacy nor the Hartman and Fithian book lists the term *desire* in its index.

Immediate Successes That May Not Last

One of the many couples who participated in a treatment experience based on the Hartman and Fithian approach had been married for almost 10 years but had not consummated the marriage. Treatment apparently had been successful; the couple had consummated the marriage and the wife had been able to experience orgasm several times toward the end of the program. They happily returned home.

About a year later the wife appeared at the treatment center, distraught and almost incoherent. Apparently, the couple had learned to handle the technical and physiological aspects of sex, but they did not know how to cope with the emotional aspects of it. It might be that by focusing so much on the physical and technical aspects of successful intercourse, insufficient attention was given to the reasons the couple had waited so long to consummate their marriage. What were all the underlying factors for insufficient desire within the partners? The communication difficulties experienced by the couple prior to treatment had not found resolution afterward; in fact, a deep distrust of the husband had developed in the wife.

Applications of Master and Johnson's and Fithian and Hartman's Work

The present author from her own training experience has come to appreciate the benefits of intensive treatment, not only for clients who have sexual difficulties but also for those with a variety of other kinds of problems. During a 1-year clinical internship at the University of Kentucky Medical School in the psychiatry department under the direction of Maxie C. Maultsby, M.D., the founder of Rational Behavior Therapy, the author was trained and supervised in the application of 1-week, 2-week, and 3-week intensive treatment programs in addition to regular weekly scheduled treatment sessions. The intense focus on the issue and its solution helped to shorten the time it often takes to come to the root of a problem. In this setting there is not much space for distraction from the work at hand.

Unfortunately, this type of therapy is a costly undertaking for the clients; they have to stay away from home and work for a week or two at a time while living in a motel. The rent for the motel accommodations, of course, does not include the costs for the treatment. At the time of publication of their book, Hartman and Fithian (1974) stated that the costs for their 2-week intensive program with a 2-year follow-up service came to $2,400.00. One can only guess what the cost would be today, more than 30 years later.

Irene: Graduate of Intensive Treatment Approaches

As women's orgasms received more attention in the public opinion in the late 1970s, Irene's husband became concerned about Irene's inability to reach orgasm. He felt it was something he should be able to provide, and they sought therapy using the Masters and Johnson approach. It did not work for them; Irene, first introduced in Chapter 4, could not get to the point of arousal that would lead to orgasm. Disappointed, they returned home and made follow-up arrangements with a local psychiatrist, who in due time used the term *frigid* to describe Irene's sexual condition.

With her marriage dissolved, still non-orgasmic, and bearing the psychiatrist's label of frigid, she gave intensive therapy one more try, although she did not have a sexual partner at the time. She had never masturbated and—due to her upbringing—her general views of sex were rather conservative. The concept of self-pleasuring provided an entry into Irene's mental and emotional reluctance to become sexual. After intensive work introducing her to self-pleasuring and the use of fantasy, Irene appeared one morning at the therapist's office with the exclamation, "I did it, I did it!" She was so excited, the words just jumped out of her mouth. Irene had experienced her first orgasm while masturbating.

When asked about the details that had been useful to her in achieving orgasm, Irene hesitated, obviously embarrassed, but she continued with her report, relating that a particular fantasy had been helpful. Her fantasy had involved a rape situation. It was difficult for this gentle woman to admit that imagining herself being raped had brought her to orgasm. Being raped meant that she did not have to accept responsibility for the sex act or her feelings in it.

Her conservative upbringing came to mind as a reason for her reluctance to assume responsibility for any sexual behavior on her part. While this was true to an extent, it was only part of the explanation. The major part came from the physical deformity she had grown up with. In her mind, in order to be a sexual—and perhaps even seductive—person, one had to be flawlessly beautiful. Women with physical defects had no business presenting themselves as sexual. They had no choices; if someone chose them, even if it was a rapist, they had to accept it because they had no other opportunities.

Irene had married the first man who asked her to and had given birth to several children. Later she was able to undergo corrective surgery, but even the surgery did not erase Irene's memories of her defect. Actually, she chose to regard the scars from the surgery as constant reminders of her imperfection. In therapy, Irene was eventually able to let go of these reminders and enjoy her body without feeling that she was barely worth the attention of a rapist. She set up new criteria for regarding her body and how she wanted to be treated.

Irene developed a curiosity that she had not allowed herself to indulge in during her adolescence and young adulthood. Along with the curiosity came a healthy interest in sexual activity. When her youngest child reached college age (the others had gone already), Irene left her hometown, moved to another state, and began training for a new profession. In her new environment, she met a man with whom she became involved in a satisfying sexual relationship. Feeling free to make choices, instead of waiting to be picked as second-best by a man, she decided to make a commitment to this relationship. Her sexual desire grew as she became free to choose with whom to have sex and when.

Adaptations of the Masters and Johnson Approach

Arentewicz and Schmidt (1983) have adopted the Masters and Johnson treatment approach with some modifications and extensions for treatment application in Germany. In their opinion, lack of desire and sexual aversion do not constitute sexual dysfunctions, although their occurrences are significant descriptive characteristics of the individuals with sexual difficulties. The German clinicians caution that in some rare cases lack of desire does not necessarily have a dysfunctional effect on sexual activity because the affected individuals may become aroused and reach orgasm. But these orgasms may be experienced as mechanical and unsatisfying to the point that the individuals may block their feelings toward their partners and develop an emotional distance from them. This finding might serve as an explanation of the events that occurred in the situation of the two spouses who had not consummated their marriage in almost 10 years before they approached treatment, as described earlier.

In their pilot study, which lasted from January 1972 to October 1973, Arentewicz and Schmidt reported treating 23 couples, using a therapist team in two sessions per week. Following this, they revised their treatment protocol and started a treatment project in Hamburg, Germany, involving 262 couples. For 5 years, psychotherapists of different backgrounds participated in the project, including physicians, psychiatrists, and psychologists trained in different theoretical treatment approaches.

Arentewicz and Schmidt: Descriptive Characteristics Among Sexual Dysfunctions

In their treatment approach, Arentewicz and Schmidt found it helpful to distinguish between several descriptive characteristics among the sexual dysfunctions. A *primary* dysfunction means that the difficulty has existed from the start of sexual relations, whereas *secondary* dysfunctions are difficulties that are noted after a symptom-free period. *Initial* dysfunctions coincide with the individual's first sexual experiences.

Difficulties that occur only in particular forms of sexual activity (for instance, coitus versus masturbation) are called *technique-related* difficulties. *Partner-related* dysfunctions are difficulties that might occur with one partner but not with another. A woman may feel interested in sex with a lover but not with the husband. *Situational* dysfunctions are those that occur only in certain situations. For instance, a couple might feel less interested in sex during their regular life, but suddenly perk up during a vacation. In addition, the severity of the complaint can be described in terms of frequency and permanence, finally with the *duration of disturbance* being another useful descriptive characteristic. Both the partner-related and the situational dysfunction types are especially relevant to women's sexual complaints.

The Hamburg Model: Changes in Problem Presentations

The treatment project in Hamburg, Germany, mentioned above, has been operating since the early 1970s as the Centre for Sex Counseling at the Department for Sex Research, University Clinic of Hamburg. It functions as a treatment facility and also trains and supervises therapists (Hauch, 1998). Compared with past years, the center has recently seen a dramatic change in the people seeking consultation. Many more women now initiate treatment and with different kinds of problems. As reported earlier, in the years between 1975 and 1977, a total of 80% of the women treated complained of lack of arousal and orgasm and 12% of vaginismus, while 67% of the men reported erectile dysfunction and 29% related ejaculation problems, complaints that were considered to be the classical sexual dysfunctions.

Quite a change was observed during the years from 1992 to 1994, when the proportion of female patients diagnosed as experiencing sexual dysphoria, or lack of sexual desire, increased from 8% to almost 60%, while the proportion of arousal and orgasm problems were reduced to 29%.

Like their counterparts in the United States, the clientele of the Hamburg center includes a significant number of women who are able to reach orgasm by manipulation or petting or intercourse but experience little or no desire to have sex with their partners. In the author's opinion, this lack of sexual desire is quite different from the classical sexual dysfunctions where symptoms develop as a result of unconscious processes. The lack of sexual desire has been viewed as "a kind of protest by these women against their partners' expectations and their own internalized norms. The underlying conflicts are more or less preconscious" (Hauch, 1998, p. 238).

The therapy basis for the Hamburg model is still the principle adapted from Masters and Johnson that the couple is the treatment unit; it is not just the partner with the symptom, emphasizing that the symptom-free partner is not to be considered as a sort of co-therapist. There are different settings in which couples therapy can be carried out. *Compact* therapy occurs over a period of 3 weeks with daily sessions conducted by two therapists (one male, one female). Following this intensive treatment, the couple is seen again in follow-up sessions 3 months and 1 year later.

The *extended* therapy schedule includes one or two sessions per week. While the treatment in this setting can be conducted by one therapist, it is considered to be beneficial if the therapist is of the same sex as the partner with the symptom. Therapy with this schedule usually requires between 40 and 60 sessions, extending over a time period of 9 to 15 months.

In the *group couples* therapy setting, three to five couples and two therapists of different sexes work in sessions that last about 3 hours on a weekly basis, extending over about 9 months and including 20 to 30 sessions. Although the group couples setting had been beneficial, recently the effort necessary to organize it has reduced some of its appeal.

While in the early years the Hamburg model incorporated many of the exercises developed by Masters and Johnson to facilitate the partners' moving closer to one another, there has been a change based on the different ways men and women respond to prevailing gender roles. A more even balance between approaching and keeping one's distance has been adopted, "encouraging both partners to develop more autonomy in their relationship on one hand, but also towards the pressures of the prevailing discourse on heterosexual normality on the other hand" (Hauch, 1998, p. 242).

Hauch (1998) cautioned therapists not to be seduced into becoming associated with a "pro-sex" position and to avoid the misperception that couples therapy is a program to teach people effective sexual techniques. Undue emphasis on exercises and techniques might lead to neglecting the deeper meaning of the clients' request, which is reflected in the symptoms. The symptoms are clients' ways of coping with underlying conflicts. It is those conflicts that need to be dealt with, making the symptoms superfluous and enabling the couple to resolve the conflict.

Alternate Models of Sex Therapy

As elements of the Masters and Johnson model were difficult to implement in typical therapeutic practice, alternate models of sex therapy have been proposed. Major changes included the utilization of a single therapist instead of a two-person therapy team and replacing the intensive treatment periods with weekly to semi-weekly sessions. In order to rule out or determine whether physiological reasons might be contributing to the sexual dysfunction, clients were instructed to schedule examinations with their own physicians (McCarthy, Ryan, & Johnson, 1975). The early alternate models maintained Masters and Johnson's notion that the complaint is a couple's problem that is not restricted to one of the partners in the relationship.

Sex enhancement exercises—including those developed by Masters and Johnson as well as modifications of them—remained as the main focus of the treatment process. Between sessions, the telephone was used to monitor the process. Apparently, 10 to 15 sessions after the assessment phase constituted the period of treatment.

The non-pharmaceutical approaches to the treatment of sexual complaints discussed here are only a few of many different treatment models and approaches available. The intensive treatment modalities that were popular a few decades ago have had to change their format, as they could not be continued due to financial considerations. In many cases, sex therapy is now incorporated into centers that are equipped to handle other psychotherapeutic situations. In other words, sex therapy as a specialty may be included with other areas within a general therapy practice or center.

Sex Therapy Within the General Psychotherapy Framework

As sex therapy has become an accepted treatment modality for problems that had previously been dealt with but not always successfully resolved with traditional insight-oriented therapies, the mental health field has seen an increase in sex therapy approaches, often within the context of general psychotherapy (Halgin, Hennessey, Statlender, Feinman, & Brown, 1988).

Perhaps the intensive treatment approaches of Masters and Johnson and Fithian and Hartman, which stretched over periods of 2 to 3 weeks, have led to the notion that sexual problems can be resolved in a short period of time and therefore, sex therapy seemed to include the promise of being a time-efficient approach. Clients may attribute difficulties arising from relational conflicts to sexual tension just as they may tend to explain sexual difficulties by citing relational conflicts.

A woman's difficulty with experiencing orgasm may be due to an underlying conflict about losing control or avoiding intimacy rather than from inadequate arousal techniques.

Most therapists recognize that relational conflicts and sexual dysfunction seldom exist independently of one another. These complaints are intertwined and it is for the therapist to decide where to intervene and provide help first—the relational or the sexual area. Often the relational aspects need to be addressed before sex therapy can begin. Instead of a narrow specialist approach therapists with a broad-based knowledge foundation would be better equipped to make those decisions. Before embarking on sex therapy, it is crucial to investigate the possible organic etiology of the complaint and it is equally critical to evaluate contributing psychological factors (Halgin et al., 1988).

Current Approaches

Suggestions for treating hypoactive sexual desire in non-pharmaceutical ways that one can find in the relevant literature include the encouragement of erotic responses through self-stimulation and arousing fantasies, reduction of anxiety with appropriate information and sensate focus exercises, enhancement of sexual experiences through improved communication and skills in initiating and refusing sexual activity, expansion of the repertoire of affectionate and sexual activities, and setting aside more time for enjoyable couple activities (LoPiccolo & Friedman, 1988).

Self-Help Books and Exercises

As an example, a slim book, covering general and specific exercises, *Sexual Exercises for Women* (Harris, 1985) promises to be the ideal manual for modern women. The author explains that sexual exercises, as a form of autosexuality, are not to be confused with masturbation. Masturbation often includes fantasy and is genital and quite different from sexual exercises, which are holistic in nature. Stressing the intimate nature of the sexual exercises, the author suggests that women engage in them when alone in order to be able to "feel truly relaxed and uninhibited" (p. 9).

In addition, there are many books on the market for women and for couples addressing a wide variety of sexual issues and providing lists of exercises and techniques designed to enhance women's sexual enjoyment and to enrich couples' sexual experiences (Berman, Berman, & Bumiller, 2001; Berman, Berman, & Schweiger, 2005; Cervenka, 2003; Ellison, 2000; Foley et al., 2002; McCarthy & MacCarthy, 2003; Zoldbrod & Dockett, 2002). Many of these books could be of great help to couples at the beginning of their relationship before resentment and bitterness have eroded the intimacy and mutual trust. Without the trust, individuals often find it difficult or embarrassing to engage in these exercises.

Additionally, some professionals caution that "sexual therapy is built upon an ongoing professional contact between the therapist and his clients. The supportive and instructional functions of the therapist cannot be achieved by a book" (McCarthy, Ryan, & Johnson, 1975). The concerns expressed by the professionals of the Hamburg model regarding sexual exercises and techniques mentioned earlier (Hauch, 1998) also deserve consideration here.

In general, the exercises require a significant level of trust in the partners. After several years of disappointments, few partners still have that type of trust and goodwill to risk such an emotional and physical exposure. Often they feel too vulnerable and awkward to embark upon such an experience. It might prove beneficial to maintain a healthy balance between closeness and autonomy, as suggested earlier (Hauch, 1998). Periods of couples or individual therapy would be indicated before recommending participation in some of these exercises.

In addition, for many women who are physically and mentally exhausted at the end of their busy days when they can finally consider sexual activities, exercises require time and energy at some point in their daily lives that they may not feel is available to them. They are faced with the choice of adding another chore to their list, thereby increasing their already high stress levels, or refusing to engage in the exercises and feeling guilty for not having done what they were supposed to do. Either way, it is not a situation likely to improve their feelings toward themselves or their partners. Therapists who incorporate suggestions for exercises in their treatment approach need to be sensitive to the couples' situations and the requirements and responsibilities in the couples' lives.

Contemporary Therapy: Treatment Approaches

There are different treatment approaches to sex therapy, and many of them have several common elements. The PLISSIT model (Annon, 1974) consists of four levels of therapy; each one providing treatment at an increasingly deeper level. PLISSIT is an acronym for these four levels: *permission, limited information, specific suggestions,* and *intensive therapy.* Giving individuals permission to appreciate their desires without comparing themselves to others is the function of the first level.

At the "limited information" level, the second level, therapists provide clients with information specific to their sexual concerns. At times factual information can alleviate anxiety and problems related to lack of knowledge. At the third level, specific suggestions cover activities and "homework" exercises that therapists recommend to clients to help them reach a goal.

The fourth, intensive therapy level can be chosen from various therapy approaches available. In *insight-oriented therapy,* or psychosexual therapy, the therapist provides interpretation and reflection to facilitate clients' awareness and understanding of unconscious feelings and thoughts that may have contributed to sexual difficulties. Another choice for the intensive therapy is the *Systems Therapy* approach. This approach is based on the concept that the problems identified are serving important current functions in the relationship. For example, a woman's low sexual desire might be an unconscious response to a perceived need to maintain a personal distance from her partner.

Postmodern sex therapy can be seen as an integration of systems, psychosexual, and behavioral approaches (LoPiccolo, 2000). Most of these behavioral approaches are designed to reduce anxiety, enhance communication, and teach new, arousal-enhancing behaviors.

There is also EMDR, eye movement desensitization and reprocessing (Shapiro, 1995). In this approach the client is directed to move his or her eyes back and forth following the movements of the therapist's fingers while the client is thinking about the problem. Apparently, this is thought to stimulate rapid and helpful informational and emotional processing in the brain similar to that which occurs during REM sleep. This approach appeared effective in alleviating persistent symptoms that had been the results of past trauma, but therapists have expanded its use to other problems, including sexual difficulties (Koehler, Zangwill, & Lotz, 2000).

Facing the Complexities of the Complaint

The list of factors influencing a woman's sense of sexual well-being or sexual vulnerability is long. Women's choices, prompted by intra-personal as well as family-of-origin factors, are determinants of their sexual attitudes and behaviors. Fears about unwanted pregnancy or sexually transmitted diseases as well as emotional reactions to infertility all can interfere with sexual desire and sexual arousal. Sexual abuse and assault, both in childhood and in adulthood, can greatly interfere with a woman's sexuality.

Childhood sexual abuse has the greatest negative impact of any childhood experience on adult sexual functioning (Courtois, 2000). Women with a history of childhood sexual abuse are two to four times more likely than other women to complain of chronic pelvic pain (Reiter & Milburn, 1994) and to experience depression, anxiety, and low self-esteem. Sexual abuse survivors report specific aversion reactions to exactly what was done to them during the sexual assault (Courtois). Sexual assault in adulthood can leave a woman with long-lasting effects. Sexual problems persisting for more than 3 years after the assault were reported by 60% of rape victims (Becker & Kaplan, 1991).

Unresolved relationship problems can be another source of sexual difficulties. Lack of trust or respect, resentment over past hurts—real or imagined—poor sexual skills, too much dependence, a partner's emotional aloofness, ineffective communication, and an imbalance of power and control—all can affect sexual interest and responsiveness. Some sex therapists (Foley, Kope, & Sugrue, 2002) consider a troubled relationship as the most common psychological cause for lack of sexual desire in women who previously experienced a normal level of sexual desire. Difficulties with sexual functioning can occur in any of the phases of the sexual response cycle. However, because sexual desire is the most frequently encountered difficulty, the remainder of this book is devoted to complaints and treatment experiences that are relevant to the desire phase of the sexual response process.

All these factors combine for an extremely complicated scenario as the backdrop for women's sexual interest and activity. The complexity of these situations in different relationships significantly affects any attempts of resolution through therapy. Focusing on the behavioral sexual aspects first may bring some short-lived successes if both partners are looking for improvement. However, the deeper issues, if not resolved, will rise to the surface again and will leave disappointed participants in the therapy process with the feeling that "it didn't work."

The Psychiatrist's Reactions

In the general context of treatment, it is interesting to learn about one psychiatrist's reactions to working with couples complaining of low sexual desire (Polonsky, 1997). It is a frustrating task to single out deeply buried conflicts and issues that appear almost impossible to resolve. The frustration of the therapist in this case seems to mirror the pain and sense of hopelessness of the clients. Initial excitement when it appears that some point of engagement has been reached often is followed by disappointment and frustration when the therapist realizes that the hoped-for breakthrough did not occur and the situation between the partners did not change.

Polonsky (1997) conceptualized the marital dynamics in the therapy situation within the object-relations perspective and in particular focused on three elements. The *repetition compulsion* is a tendency to repeat behavioral patterns that result in pain and suffering. Early learned patterns developed in the individual's family of origin may be reenacted in the current relationship. In the author's opinion, low sexual desire often has its origin in the early object relationships.

For the repetition compulsion to work, couples have to collude in a reciprocal way. *Collusion* occurs when one spouse has an "overt" sexual problem while the other is the complaining (or silent) deprived partner. A change in the overt difficulty may reveal the hidden discomforts of the spouse in the therapy process and treatment is sabotaged.

Mutual projections and *projective identifications* constitute the third element. In this complicated process hated parts of the self are projected onto the spouse, where they then may be criticized. Through this progression, the perception of the spouse is transformed and interactions and communications transpire through the filter of the family of origin. What is intended by one person is different from the way it is perceived by the other, and these misperceptions may camouflage clients' resistance to change, at times creating confusion and frustration in the therapist.

Polonsky (1997) compared the therapy process to a marriage: there is initial excitement because this is something new and seems to hold promise. There may be enough energy in the honeymoon phase that suggestions are followed by the clients, allowing for some apparent change to occur. But when the old difficulties reemerge, the therapist begins to experience feelings that reflect the frustrations and disappointments that the couple has gone through. It is important to remember that the need for a given symptom and the importance of not relinquishing it is often not considered or accepted by therapists. Low desire might function to maintain a balance in some couples' lives.

Another Psychiatrist's Response

In his response to Dr. Polonsky, psychiatrist Stephen Levine (1997) stated, "Low sexual desire states are invitations for our investigatory skills. These problems do not lend themselves to technology for solutions" (p. 17). Instead, Levine suggested engaging in a process of respectful investigation, analyzing the main factors that have impacted the couple's (or person's) sexual potential and helping clients to assume responsibility for the contributing causes as well as thinking more clearly about factors that did not cause the problem and may be available as helpful alternatives.

Theoretical Orientation

Among the various theoretical approaches available, which ones lend themselves to "respectful investigation" mentioned above by Levine? Surveys of American psychologists, Canadian psychologists, and Canadian counselors about theoretical orientation and influential theorists (Warner, 1991) have shown a preference for an eclectic orientation. Cognitive-behavioral theory was the second choice for Canadian psychologists and third choice for Canadian counselors and American psychologists. Albert Ellis (rational-emotive behavior therapy) and Carl Rogers (person-centered therapy) were named among the top three as the most influential contemporary therapists. American psychologists included Sigmund Freud (psychoanalytic therapy) in the top three and gave psychoanalytic theory second place. Aaron Beck (cognitive therapy) was named by the other two groups as one of the top three influential therapists.

Another survey inquiring about counseling approaches utilized in group therapy by certified alcohol and drug counselors and counselor trainees in the state of Arkansas revealed that most adhered to Reality Therapy. Behavior Therapy was second in preference, and Rational Emotive Therapy and Rogerian approaches tied for third place (Whisnant, Hammond, & Tilmon, 1999).

More recently, cognitive-behavioral approaches appear to have achieved greater popularity. In general, cognitive therapy works on the principle that people make purposeful behavioral decisions, based on a wide range of choices, but do not always choose the most self-enhancing one. In therapy, clients have opportunities to reexamine those choices and learn a new way of thinking and decision-making. Different decisions result in different behaviors and different feelings. Clients are encouraged to identify, challenge, and reject (if appropriate) old beliefs. And even though new ways of behaving may be less than perfect, individuals can free themselves from repeating the same behaviors and expecting different and better results (Maass, & Neely, 2000).

Many therapists working within a cognitive-behavioral framework assume that people's belief systems are triggered by environmental influences and people's thoughts about them. A concurrent assumption holds that people act as if their perceptions are accurate and their beliefs are true. Beliefs are the major components of attitudes about situations, other people, and values that include goals, morals, and ethics.

Following initial attempts at identifying problem areas and exploring "solutions" that did not resolve problems, attention is focused on teaching clients the connection between their thoughts and beliefs that lead to dysfunctional behavior and negative emotional consequences. Those beliefs become the targets of intervention—where did they come from? How did they influence previous behaviors? Did the behavior result in positive or negative consequences? If the consequences were negative, can beliefs be modified and thus lead to different behaviors with better outcomes?

Aaron Beck (1976) recognized that cognitive therapy and psychoanalysis are insight therapies. Both address thoughts, feelings, and wishes that clients report. In its problem-solving approach, which includes clients as active participants, cognitive therapy deals with consciously derived meanings and inferences that are available to the client for consideration and correction. Cognitive therapists seek to understand the elements of how clients misinterpret reality, rather than to find out why they do so.

The following chapter will outline and address in detail cognitive-behavioral factors that are relevant to the treatment of clients complaining of reduced or absent sexual desire.

9
Cognitive-Behavioral Factors Relevant to Treatment

The previous chapter, along with describing early ground-laying efforts in sexology and sex therapy, also outlined the complexity of contributing factors facing therapists when working with clients on issues of sexual desire. Connected to all the contributing factors are cognitive elements that clients at times are not aware of. Yet these cognitive elements are instrumental in shaping the person's attitudes about each contributing factor. The attitudes can be of a positive or negative nature, enhancing or interfering, depending on the person's evaluation of the particular issue.

Aaron T. Beck (1988), professor of psychiatry and proclaimed father of Cognitive Therapy, described the essence of couples' cognitive therapy as consisting "of exploring with troubled partners their unrealistic expectations, self-defeating attitudes, unjustified negative explanations, and illogical conclusions" (p. 14). Explorations of partners' ways of drawing conclusions about each other and their particular patterns of communicating with each other often shed light on misperceptions and misunderstandings that have led to troubled situations and provide guidance for more reasonable, less hostile interactions.

Cognitive Interference in Sexual Excitement

Instead of focusing on erotic thoughts during sexual interactions, individuals may distract themselves with negative thoughts that will eventually lead to decreased subjective and physiological arousal and to difficulties in both males and females. In males, these cognitive distractions are usually related to erection concerns, anticipating failure and negative consequences. Cognitive interference in the sexual response process in women results mainly from focusing on negative thoughts about physical attractiveness (Dove & Wiederman, 2000). As with many other behavioral aspects, there is a direct link between cognition and emotions and their subsequent impact on sexual functioning.

Feedback Model of Sexual Arousal

More than two decades ago a conception of the sexual arousal cycle, which emphasized the cognitive elements that are involved in human sexual functioning, was proposed (Walen, 1980). This conception featured a feedback model with eight links arranged in a chain where each of the links serves as a cue for the next link and—at the same time—as a reinforcer for the preceding link. In this model, links 1 and 2 consist of the perception of a sexual stimulus and the evaluation of that stimulus. The third link would be the physiological arousal with links 4 and 5 constituting the perception of the arousal and the evaluation of the arousal and its perception. Then some type of sexual behavior follows. The perception of that sexual behavior and the evaluation of the behavior make up links 7 and 8. Thus, in this chain, links 1, 2, 4, 5, 7, and 8 are cognitive operations—subjective perceptions and evaluations.

Tracing the process of the model, we can imagine the following scene: One of the partners in a couple initiates sexual activity. The other partner perceives the initiation as subjectively irritating and evaluates it with a thought like "I am too tired and want to go to sleep." At link 3 there may not be much or any physiological arousal, which the person perceives at link 4 and evaluates it (link 5) as "I am not in the mood; I'm not getting anything out of this!" If under these circumstances sexual behavior continues at link 6, the perception and evaluation of that behavior at links 7 and 8 will most likely be negative, even if the physiological experience was not as negative because the person may have become sufficiently aroused to experience an orgasm.

Because every link in the chain reinforces the preceding event, at link 2 the negative subjective perception is reinforced with the negative evaluation of "I am too tired," which, in turn, serves as the cue for not becoming subjectively aroused. Links 4 and 5, "I am not in the mood; I'm not getting anything out of this!" reinforce the negativity of link 3 and set the stage for more negativity in the following links.

Walen (1980) suggested that instead of emphasizing sexual behaviors, sex therapy should focus more directly on the emotional disturbance and the negative, non-playful attitudes of the individual because these cognitive factors function as significant impediments to sexual enjoyment. Walen's conception may have been a suggestion to follow Kaplan (1979) and move from sex therapy to "psychosexual therapy."

The Concept of Modes

Previously, cognitive theories have emphasized the importance of thought processing mediating emotional and behavioral responses. More recently though, Beck (1996) has proposed a different concept based on a network of interdependent cognitive, emotional, and behavioral dimensions—termed *modes*.

Modes are thought of as specific subsystems or sub-organizations made up of cognitive, emotional, and behavioral elements within a person's personality organization. The various subsystems of cognitive, affective, and behavioral parts provide schemas or scenarios within which the person will most likely respond to different situations and experiences. For instance, a person who feels depressed would have thoughts of loss or disappointment and would have the behavioral tendency to withdraw.

Cognitive Schemas and Levels Of Cognitive Interference

Based on this theoretical background, Nobre and Pinto-Gouveia (2003) developed measures to evaluate the roles and interactions between thought processes and the related emotions within the area of sexual functioning. In addition to the Sexual Modes Questionnaire (SMQ), which focuses on the connection between cognitive and emotional variables and sexual responses, the researchers constructed measures to study different levels of cognitive interference (sexually dysfunctional beliefs) and cognitive schemas. A total of 456 subjects (201 females and 255 males) were recruited for the study.

The results demonstrated that for the female subjects the greater the degree of negative thoughts occurring during sexual activity, the greater the likelihood of experiencing negative emotions and the less likely the tendency to feel pleasure and satisfaction. Similarly for the male sample, a higher degree of negative thoughts elicited greater levels of disillusionment, sadness, and shame and produced less of a tendency to feel satisfied and pleasured.

In the Sexual Modes Questionnaire, the items for the *female version* tapped six different factors: (1) Sexual Abuse Thoughts, (2) Failure and Disengagement Thoughts, (3) Partner's Lack of Affection, (4) Sexual Passivity and Control, (5) Lack of Erotic Thoughts, and (6) Low Self-Body-Image. In the *male version* of the questionnaire items were grouped around five factors: (1) Failure Anticipation and Catastrophizing Thoughts, (2) Erection Concern Thoughts, (3) Age- and Body-Function-Related Thoughts, (4) Negative Thoughts Toward Sex, and (5) Lack of Erotic Thoughts.

Examples of negative thoughts in the Failure and Disengagement category of the female version are "I'm not getting turned on" or "When will this be over?" The Partner's Lack of Affection factor was expressed in thoughts, such as "He is not as affectionate as he used to be" or "He only loves me if I am good in bed" or "This way of having sex is immoral." The Sexual Abuse category contained thoughts that sex therapists are familiar with: "Sex is all he thinks about." "He is violating me." "This is disgusting." "I have other more important matters to deal with." "How can I get out of this situation?" "If I refuse to have sex, he will cheat on me." The category of Low Self-Body-Image thoughts included "I'm getting fat/ugly" and "I'm not as physically attractive as I used to be." Again, these are statements often heard by sex therapists.

Heather: Women's Contribution to What They Experience as Abuse

The sadness inherent in these thought processes is that some women, by allowing their bodies to be part of sexual encounters that they don't enjoy, may be gradually contributing to what they experience as abuse. Heather was sexually inexperienced when she met Doug, but she was relatively open-minded and enjoyed their sexual activities during the early years of their marriage. With time, Doug was not satisfied with their sex life; he desired more stimulating sex play and acting-out fantasies. He first requested and then demanded that Heather talk in vulgar language and that she express wishes to have sex with other men; sometimes it was a friend or neighbor, at other times it might be an actor they had seen in a movie or on TV. Heather did not enjoy this behavior, but because she wanted to please Doug, she went along with it. Slowly the thoughts about her own feelings were replaced with concentrating in her mind on what Doug wanted and how she might be able to overcome her distaste for what she was doing.

However, as Doug's demands escalated to the point where she suspected that he really wanted her to have sex with another man while he was watching them, her fearful thoughts kept her from feeling the once pleasurable sensations in her body and she came to dread sex. She experienced the cognitive conflict of wanting to please Doug but at the same time being fearful of what he might demand of her next. What she once had been able to enjoy was now something she feared. She finally confronted Doug with her suspicion but because she had been compliant for so long, he refused to believe she was sincere in not wanting to continue acting out some of his fantasies.

Many women who consider men to be not only the initiators but also the leaders in sexual activity hesitate to express their own wishes and try to guess what their partners expect of them. As we know, guesswork includes opportunities for being incorrect. If we don't check out the correctness of our guesses, we can go on indefinitely acting on assumptions and beliefs that have no basis in reality. Similarly, those who think that their partners demonstrate less affectionate sexual behaviors may have paved the way by cutting short foreplay activities and encouraging their partners to "hurry up" in order to get it over with. When the partner follows the spoken or unspoken "hurry up" directions, some degree of affection gets cut out.

Thoughts like those mentioned in the Sexual Modes Questionnaire above are frequently found in the minds of women with low sexual desire. When women think of being abused in sexual activities, they feel accordingly. By categorizing these thoughts as expressing a sexual abuse factor, the researchers have indicated the intensity of dislike the women experience in those situations. With strong negative emotions like these, which are reinforced and intensified every time the woman is confronted with the possibility of sexual interaction, it is not surprising that she attempts to prolong the periods between sexual intercourse and to shorten the time spent in actual sexual activities.

As outlined previously, thoughts from the abusive category elicit intense dislike and anger in the women who comply with undesired sexual activities. Low self-image thoughts, on the other hand, primarily lead to fear and anxiety as the woman anticipates being critically judged for her physical shortcomings and possibly being abandoned for a younger, more attractive rival. Many women practice body surveillance—constantly watching and examining their bodies for any flaws—as well as self-comparison with other women. Their cognitive vigilance in both these areas serves to reinforce their body dissatisfaction (McKinley, 2002). It also invades every aspect of their sexual activity.

The Anxiety-Relief-Anxiety Cycle

For those women who do not find sex exciting for its own sake, their already weakened motivation will not be sufficient to sustain them through an evening of passionate sex after a full day's work. There is no time or inclination for romance, no time to build up excitement or arousal when one is already tired. Because of their negative anticipation they can't think of much pleasure during sexual inter-action, and many women put it off as long as they can without the risk of divorce. When they finally agree to it, they encourage their men to proceed to the sex act without a lot of foreplay just to "get it over with." Without romance and play, sex ceases to be lovemaking and becomes just another dreaded chore to perform—as in the cases of Lynn and Claire—and finally leads to the "negative anticipation and relief when it's over" cycle.

As shown in Table 9.1 below, it is a vicious cycle which starts with *anxiety* and dread about having to participate in sex. As the days pass between sexual activi-ties, the anxiety mounts; headaches may develop and give rise to the hope that the husband—observing his wife's suffering—will not persist in his requests for sex. But the anxiety steadily increases until finally the woman makes the decision to engage in sex, which she will not enjoy because she hurries the man along in

TABLE 9.1. Anxiety-Relief-Anxiety Cycle

Day	Thoughts	Feelings	Actions
1			Intercourse
2	I'm glad it's over (last night).	Relief, relaxed	None
3	No worry about sex; don't think about it.	Good, relaxed	None
4	I wonder when he'll start pushing again.	Slightly anxious	None
5	He is looking at me in that way.	Anxiety rising	None
6	He tried to touch me while I was cooking. He'll probably try harder after dinner.	Moderate anxiety	None, Refused
7	He was grumpy after I turned him down.	Strong anxiety	None
8	He has a cold and made no attempts at sex. I'll be safe for a couple of days.	Reduced anxiety, sympathy	None
9	His cold is not as bad as I thought.	Moderate anxiety	None
10	Here we go again. I am so anxious. I can't go through with it. He should know that I don't feel good enough. He should not pressure me so.	High anxiety, anger, possible explosiveness	None Refused
11	Last night was a bad scene. I'm not up to it, but I can't put it off any longer.	Extreme anxiety, guilt, anger, depression, Relief, relaxed	Intercourse
12	Well, we did it. I didn't feel much. At least, it's over for a while.	Relief, relaxed	None

Beginning of New Cycle

order to get it over with. Then she allows herself the feeling of relief because she does not have to worry about it (but in reality she does worry) for another week or so. This process resembles the dynamics that operate in the development and maintenance of phobias (Maass, 2002). Although the cycle includes some good feelings, they are not due to an enjoyable experience, but because the dreaded situation is over—at least, for the moment. The feelings of relief, in turn, reinforce the notion that the situation was indeed dreadful, thereby adding another layer to the anxiety-relief-anxiety cycle.

What can break the cycle? A change in women's attitudes not only about themselves as sexual beings, but also about deciding and planning to set the stage for them to be successful at it. It takes a resolution for women to discontinue automatically doing things they do not enjoy doing. Before participating in an activity, women might investigate the reasons for disliking what they are expected to do and to explore the possibilities of incorporating pleasure and enjoyment into the activity. The long-standing belief that women have to perform as expected by the world around them is ripe for a challenge. It is time to change the mindset from a purpose-driven motivation to a more pleasure-oriented motivation. If men are able to do it, why shouldn't women be able to think this way?

Indeed, the woman could start by evaluating the aftermath of her sexual interaction in different, perhaps more honest, terms. Was sex really that awful or were there moments that could be considered pleasing if she had been relaxed? If sex was awful, what in particular made it so? How can it be changed? If there were fleeting pleasant moments, how can they be emphasized and perhaps lengthened?

Behavioral Interactions Determining Relationship Quality and Sexual Satisfaction

The way partners interact determines in large part the quality of their relationship, and the relationship quality—in turn—affects sexual satisfaction. Clashes in interaction styles often lead to unresolved conflicts, such as one or the other partner not feeling loved, thereby creating an emotional distance (Davidson & Darling, 1988). The association of intimate communication, such as self-disclosure, with both sexual satisfaction and relationship satisfaction has been shown in past research (Cupach & Comstock, 1990). Individuals who effectively communicate their own feelings and wishes find that their self-disclosure brings them emotionally closer to their partners and increases sexual satisfaction (MacNeil & Byers, 2005). Not surprisingly, O'Leary and Arias (1983) have found that marital therapy that focused on nonsexual relationship issues resulted in significant increases in sexual satisfaction.

When leading experts on women's sexual health, (Berman, Berman, & Schweiger, 2005) briefly addressed the issue of hypoactive sexual desire disorder, they suggested that—after having ruled out physical factors—the women look at their relationships and search for ways to improve them. However, the relational aspects of sexuality are neglected by the American Psychiatric Association's

DSM (*Diagnostic and Statistical Manual of Mental Disorders*) approach, even though these aspects often lie at the root of sexual satisfactions and problems, complains The Working Group for a New View of Women's Sexual Problems (2001). "The *DSM*'s reduction of 'normal sexual function' to physiology implies, incorrectly, that one can measure and treat genital and physical difficulties without regard to the relationship in which sex occurs" (p. 3).

Women's Sexual Response Cycle

Considering the traditional model of the human sex response cycle—desire, arousal, orgasm, and resolution—to be unrealistic for describing women's sexual functioning in long-term relationships, Basson (2000) proposed a different model (see also discussion of Basson algorithm in Chapter 2). She agreed that women may relate to the traditional model at the beginning of a relationship, but over time there is a change in women's responsiveness resulting from changes in the relationship due to increased distraction and fatigue associated with increased family responsibilities. From a point of sexual neutrality, a woman might become aware of a nonsexual need for sex, which might prompt her to make a deliberate choice stimulation (perhaps thoughts, fantasies, or actual physical touch, etc.). As a consequence, some sexual arousal would develop, followed by an awareness of the wish to continue the experience for sexual reasons also. Arousal increases and may be followed by orgasm or not, but will bring a sense of physical well-being.

Basson (2000) considered factors such as emotional closeness, love, affection, acceptance, and commitment as "spin-offs" for the woman following this model. Thus, the woman is moved toward sexual experiences not necessarily by a strong biological force, but by an expectation of increased emotional closeness and a pleasant physical experience. Participation in foreplay is necessary, according to Basson, for this motivation to continue.

If we applied this model to the case of Claire and Gus discussed in Chapter 5, what changes could we anticipate? At some point Claire had mentioned that Gus was usually in a bad mood when returning home from work. Gus admitted that he was cranky because on the way home he usually thought about Claire turning him down for sex. Assuming that Claire would like Gus to be in a better mood, she might think sexual activity would accomplish that and she could make a deliberate decision to stimulate herself in ways that worked for her. Allowing Gus time for foreplay, her arousal would increase and she might want to continue with sex because it felt good to her. Most likely, she would experience orgasm—she usually did.

The following day Gus would be in a happier mood coming home and might even remember not to leave his belt, socks, and so on in different places around the house. If not, a friendly reminder at this time would probably be more successful than angry nagging. As long as Claire operated out of a framework of punishment this model would not work because she would consider her willingness to have sex as reinforcing the bad behavior, when in her opinion Gus deserved punishment. The woman operating successfully out of this model needs to have a clear conception of her own investment in the relationship.

Concurrent Changes in Relationship Satisfaction and Sexual Satisfaction

The results of a study involving 87 individuals in long-term relationships revealed that changes in relationship satisfaction did not necessarily lead to changes in sexual satisfaction or the other way around, but sexual satisfaction and relationship satisfaction were found to change concurrently (Byers, 2005). The investigator proposed that the quality of intimate communication accounted in part for the concurrent changes in relationship satisfaction and sexual satisfaction.

How do we measure the quality of intimate communication? By asking participants to rate the level of satisfaction they derive from their partner's communication? Do we question participants about what they say to each other and what their thoughts are about what they just heard or said? Seldom do we consider the various characteristics that constitute elements of communication or interaction. Although there are many books available on topics such as interpersonal communication, expression of emotions, and the awareness of how these variables influence our interactions with others, we seldom apply these factors to intimate sexual contacts within long-term committed relationships.

Behavioral Aspects: Interference in Sexual Excitement

As was demonstrated in Walen's (1980) feedback model and Beck's (1996) concept of modes as well as in the work on cognitive schemas (Nobre & Pinto-Gouveia, 2003) that developed out of Walen's and Beck's considerations, behavioral aspects are closely linked to cognitive aspects within the overall sexual response process. Behavioral aspects are influenced by their positive or negative cognitive precursors; and, in turn, the behaviors serve to reinforce the originally positive or negative cognitions.

Individual Interaction Styles

People interact with others on a daily basis. Some of their interactions proceed in an amicable, pleasant manner, while others may create feelings of sadness, disappointment, or even anger. Most of our interactions are not just one-time occurrences but rather constitute important parts of the relationships we have with others. As ingredients of relationships, interactions take on meaning in and of themselves. They become the messengers of the feelings, goals, hopes, wishes, and expectations we hold for a particular relationship.

Through their recurring nature, individual interactions over time combine into a pattern that forms a person's particular interaction style. With continued practice, the individual's pattern of interaction seems to function automatically. More often than not, people do not feel the need to pause before responding in their long-practiced way to evaluate what their goal of the interaction is and whether or not the particular interaction is conducive to achieving this goal. Before responding, people often forget to ask themselves two simple and basic questions: "What do I want?" and "How do I get it?"

Gus and Claire: The Sharp Edge of Sarcasm

One of the lessons to be learned from the case of Claire and Gus can be found in their interaction styles. When Gus was hurting emotionally he used sarcasm to hide behind. He did not want to admit the pain he experienced when he felt rejected by Claire. Unfortunately, Claire was a good match for him. She possessed her own not insignificant arsenal of sarcastic responses. It had become a competition between them that neither one could win without losing a lot. As outlined earlier in the application of the Basson model, the resolution of the sarcasm issue could be attempted in that framework also.

Interaction Style: Charisma

Some may consider interaction styles to be inherent in people's personalities or they regard individuals' interactions as expressions of a given individual's personality configuration. Are there personality constellations that appear to be more successful in social interactions than other personality profiles? People seem to think so and often explain the reason for some person's social success with the charisma this person apparently possesses.

Charismatic people appear to have successes in many of life's areas; they are successful in their careers, their marriages, and in their relationships with others. We may even detect an element of charisma in the hero of romance novels as he sweeps the heroine off her feet. Charisma functions well in the art of seduction, which plays a significant role in the early part of a relationship and, as discussed in Chapter 5, too often gets lost as the relationship develops into a long-term liaison.

Because we usually consider charisma in the general context of being spectacularly successful, we often think of it as a rare gift, bestowed upon a special few. And although the word carries the meaning "a divine gift of grace," social psychologist Ronald Riggio (1987) does not believe that it is an inherited quality, given to some people. It is something that can be developed by many of us. According to Riggio, charisma is not a single trait in a person; instead it is a constellation of different basic social skills that in combination make up a charisma potential. Sarcasm is not one of the basic social skills contributing to a person's charisma. And if we asked Claire or Gus, neither would describe the other's interaction style as charismatic.

Interaction Style: Emotional Intelligence

Recently emotional intelligence has become a popular concept in psychology (Goleman, 1995). We are told that emotional intelligence consists of a set of capabilities that are necessary for success in life—success in social interactions as well as in intimate personal relations. What exactly are the capabilities that make up emotional intelligence? How can we identify them in ourselves and in others? It has been suggested that self-knowledge consisting of an awareness of one's emotions, an ability to manage those emotions appropriately, and self-motivation provides the foundation of emotional intelligence.

Whether we talk about charisma or emotional intelligence, we tend to neglect its importance in sexual relationships. When we are the most vulnerable as in situations of physical and emotional intimacy, we often underestimate the protection provided by engaging in emotionally intelligent behaviors. What can one possibly gain by using caustic verbal expressions, such as sarcasm, ridicule, accusations, and similarly destructive verbal exchanges, in situations that are expected to lead to lovemaking? Even if low libido had not been a significant problem in the overall relationship so far, caustic verbal expressions may well have a reducing effect on libido and become a contributing factor in the development of reduced sexual desire.

It is also helpful here to remember that men and women often have different communication styles as well as different communication goals (Tannen, 1994). Women use language to promote closeness and build intimacy, whereas men use language to convey information, to challenge others, and to achieve status in a group. In talking about her concerns, a woman wants to foster a sense of sharing and she wants a response that tells her she is being understood and she is not alone. But the man in his response may go straight to offering advice or solutions.

Robert: Criticism as Emotional Intelligence?

Robert, a successful engineer in a supervisory position, reluctantly learned the connection between his criticizing verbal behavior and his wife's frequent lack of sexual desire. Monica told her side: "When Robert comes home he usually asks me or the children why we did or did not do a certain thing. He puts us on the defensive as soon as he enters the house. It could be that somebody left a toy or magazine lying around or something was broken. He always finds something."

Robert did not deny Monica's report. In fact, he admitted that he used the same approach at his job and it worked well for him. He would allow a brief time for his subordinates to defend themselves, and after that they willingly and silently went about making the changes demanded by Robert. With this strategy, Robert achieved similar results at home—except that Monica was seldom in the mood for lovemaking and his children hardly ever asked him for help with any of their projects.

Initially, Robert refused to acknowledge the link between his behavior and his wife's lack of response to sex. In his opinion, his alertness to any wrongdoings in the family was essential to their functioning; it was important to keep up the values and standards of the family. If Monica turned his vigilance into a problem in their sex life, then she was not fulfilling her part of being his helpmate. The realization that he was in a position to gain an emotionally warmer reception from his family by changing his approach to them did not come overnight. But when he finally learned to reduce and modify his criticism, he agreed that the consequences were worth the effort of heeding the lessons of emotional intelligence.

Communication During Sex

Communication during sexual activities can be arousing and stimulating to some but disturbing and embarrassing to others. Because of the silent stoic image endorsed by many men, they may find it difficult to verbalize any feelings during sex even though research has shown long ago that many women feel inhibited in their own arousal by the men's silence during sex play (DeMartino, 1970).

Women may get the impression that "nice" women are not supposed to be passionate in their expressions and so they remain just as silent as their male partners. Edith and Ruth, encountered earlier, had married unresponsive men who were not willing to experiment and try out different sexual activities; the two women also had to face silence during sexual intercourse. Neither man was given to expressions of emotions or passion. As Ruth said, "It's like he is making love to himself, not me. Sometimes I feel like an object or aid for masturbation, so that he won't need to use his hands." It is not difficult to estimate the level of resentment behind Ruth's statement.

Nonverbal Interaction Styles

Emotional intelligence not only affects individuals' verbal expressions, it is reflected in their nonverbal interactions as well. Smiles and touch can convey a range of different messages. Touch is a powerful way to convey nonverbal sexual communication. A gentle, sensuous touch transmits a different message from that of a hard powerful grip. A gentle stroke of the hand can defuse anger, whereas a grabbing motion can induce fear. Facial expressions are often a feedback mode about the impact our behavior has made upon another person. From approval to disgust, facial expressions cover a wide range of communication.

Body language can speak volumes, from the way a person turns toward or away from another, the interpersonal space or distance the individual maintains, to the body's bend and the configuration of the arms. For instance, crossed arms in front of one's chest do not indicate an invitation to come closer. To achieve emotional closeness, an intimate partnership needs to be based on a cooperative foundation with open communication, avoiding ambiguous contacts. At any particular time, the various methods of communication should convey messages of similar meaning and content.

Awareness of the Effect of One's Interaction Style

Consider for a moment a situation involving the "anxiety-relief-anxiety cycle" introduced earlier: as a woman's level of anxiety increases over days, her inter-action style may be terse if she considers her partner's wishes for sex to be an imposition, or it may be vague if she wants to delay giving in but also hopes not to offend her partner. Neither response style is designed to make her partner feel good about the relationship. If she responds in an abrupt and terse manner, he most likely will become angry and accusing in his expressions. If her style is ambiguous, her partner may resort to sarcasm in order to hide the discomfort he experiences with the woman's vague response. On day 10 of the cycle, the com-bination of feeling extremely anxious and angry may cause the woman's interac-tion style to become explosive.

Again, interactions like those are not conducive to elicit loving or accepting responses from the partner or to make both partners feel sympathetic or intimate toward each other. Thus, it would be beneficial for the woman not only to be aware of her feelings but also to know how her general interaction style is impacted by the varying emotions she experiences. Furthermore, over time, the woman will have ample opportunity to observe her partner's response to her when she is acting under the influence of her feelings. By observing and recording in her mind her partner's responses, she will be able to predict his behaviors before she decides on a way to handle the situation.

Unfortunately, many women who have little desire for sexual interaction avoid thinking about it until it becomes a pressing issue. The tendency to become frustrated with the mounting anxiety is great, often to the point where calm and clear thinking is not easily possible for the individual. Learning about one's feelings and one's way of expressing them as well as the likely reaction to that expression from others in one's environment is best accomplished in a calm state of mind.

Emotional intelligence includes capabilities or skills that are required for suc-cess in intimate personal relations. Awareness of one's emotions and an ability to manage those emotions appropriately are among those skills. Managing emotions appropriately includes an awareness of how those around us are affected by our expression of emotions. Perhaps the significance of this awareness has not been fully comprehended by some men like Tom and Fred (discussed in Chapter 5), for instance, and therefore a need for change has not become obvious to them. As long as women believe the notion of men's gender-related silence, they will tol-erate behaviors that in the end will lead to disappointment and resentment in themselves and their relationships.

Rather than accepting men's silence as their entitlement or limitation, or as a genetic factor, women would do well to teach their men the importance of open communication—including that of emotions—in intimate relationships. Preferably, that teaching will emphasize the fact that in the end men stand to win by communicating openly because they receive greater and more pleasing atten-tion from women.

In humans, all sexual activities—like all other activities—include a wide range of elements of cognition and elements of behavior accounting for the complexities of interactions. There are so many opportunities for misperceptions, miscommunications, and misunderstandings ready to upset the delicate balance of intimate interactions. Awareness and understanding of how these elements are interconnected and how we can influence the outcomes of particular interactions are tools and skills that present us with opportunities for controlling to some degree whether our interactions with significant others will be pleasant and rewarding or unpleasant and disappointing.

The "habit" of awareness can be developed by exploring the likely consequences of every one of our important decisions before acting on them. A blank copy of the Interaction Style Scale is provided in Appendix A so the reader can practice becoming aware of his or her own and other's manner of interacting.

Some professionals regard cognitive-behavioral therapy (CBT) mostly as a short-term therapeutic treatment modality to be used with a wide range of problems (Fusco & Apsche, 2005), yet all the factors explored in this chapter are significant areas that require time to explore with cognitive-behavioral approaches. Neglecting the impact of these factors and leaving them unexplored might render a treatment approach superficial.

Along with other experts in the field of CBT, Fusco and Apsche (2005) emphasize the aspect of time-limitedness when they describe CBT as "a relatively structured ... active, directive, time limited approach" (p. 76), in which the identification of clients' behavioral patterns and accompanying cognitive processes constitute the major thrust of CBT, where cognitive processes include clients' thoughts, perceptions, underlying beliefs, attributions, and so forth. "The overarching goal of CBT, therefore, is to change or alter those beliefs that have led to distress or dysfunction" (p. 76), the authors explained. Fusco and Apsche have developed their approach within the framework of Beck's schema concept (discussed earlier) with the incorporation of techniques such as relaxation, assertiveness training, and cost-benefit analysis.

The purpose of mentioning their work here is to introduce one of many current variations of the cognitive-behavioral treatment orientation. The present author, having had the privilege of being trained in the early and groundbreaking formulations of the leaders in the cognitive-emotive behavioral field, such as Rational Behavior Therapy (RBT) (Maxie C. Maultsby, Jr., M.D.) and (then) Rational Emotive Therapy (RET) (Albert Ellis, Ph.D.), has developed her own variation of treatment which is firmly based on the principles of those early scholars but incorporates a more elaborate focus on behavioral alternatives while placing an equally detailed attention on the exploration and challenging of clients' cognitive processes. This approach is described in more detail in the following chapter.

10
A Practical Cognitive-Behavioral Treatment Approach

Theorists believe that individuals have a range of behavior change opportunities to augment inner strength in their quest for doing better and feeling better. Cognitive therapists assume that faulty thinking causes psychological problems. Therefore, in developing a practical psychotherapy, their treatment plans consist of identifying aberrations in thought processes, testing the validity of thoughts and beliefs, and modifying thoughts and attitudes that lead to unrealistic evaluation and misconceptions (Maass & Neely, 2000).

Elements of the Treatment Process

Clearly defined steps that facilitate exploration of the validity of underlying beliefs, modification of beliefs where indicated, development of goals, and designation of behavioral options designed to reach them—all within a calm atmosphere—are the ingredients of this treatment approach. This approach constitutes a move away from the usual problem-focused therapy. The difference is subtle, a matter of semantics, some may say. However, it expresses a significant shift in attitudes.

Conceptualizing Challenges Instead of Problems

Clients are invited to think about issues they want to discuss as *challenges* rather than as problems because "the notion of 'challenges' evokes the idea of a stimulating, provocative, or interesting task, inviting the person to engage in efforts that lead to the task's solution. The implication is that the person has the ability to manage the task. The word *problem* on the other hand, connotes a source of perplexity or distress, something that is difficult to handle. It may even reflect on the person as being 'problematic' or incapable of coping. While the task may indeed be difficult, we want to assume that we are capable of working on resolving it" (Maass, 2002, p. 49).

Goals: Providing Direction

Implicit in the challenge is the notion of a goal. For example, when defining the challenge, clients describe the disturbing situation, such as not enjoying sexual activities. To be meaningful, the challenge needs to include a goal; otherwise the challenge remains unresolved. The goal could be conceptualized either as experiencing enjoyment while engaging in sex or—as an alternative—refraining from sex. Goals provide a purpose and give direction to the process. But goals need to be well defined and realistic in their size and scope. Unmanageable or unrealistic goals are ineffective because they lead to early discouragement and defeat.

Options and Their Probability for Success

With the therapist's guidance, background issues and the emotional components relevant to the situation will be explored. Identification of behavioral *options* and estimation of their probabilities for success are subsequent steps. The different success probabilities serve as basis for option selection; it would be logical to start with the option that contains the greatest likelihood of success and a low risk of failure.

Decisions and Actions

When a decision has been made about which option to adopt, it is time to implement action. Action includes planning on how to carry out the various steps needed to reach the goal. The action phase also includes preparations, such as behavior rehearsals and the use of mental imagery techniques—all pointing toward and culminating in the actual behaviors necessary to reach the goal and master the challenge.

Starting the Process

In the case of Claire and Gus discussed earlier, the situation had been explored and some of the options were obvious. Gus saw two options: resolving the situation with the help of therapy or divorce. Claire wanted to rule out divorce, so both had agreed on an option and started action by engaging in therapy. Following this preliminary phase, work with Claire and Gus individually as well as in conjoint sessions proceeded with initial emphasis on Claire's part. What would make sex more pleasurable for her? Claire's immediate answer was that if Gus picked up after himself, she would not have so many angry thoughts about him. It sounded like a beginning; but as long as Claire regarded sex as something that Gus wanted and she was supposed to give, Claire would still not be able to find enough pleasurable aspects in sex for herself.

Another point of interest here is that Claire immediately focused on what Gus could do differently. The tendency to focus on what the partner could or should do is a common occurrence when clients are asked what would constitute an improvement in the current situation.

Turning the discussion to what Claire could do, she expressed willingness to work on separating the old hurts from the current displeasing situations. With less anger would she be more inclined to have intimate times with Gus? She would still be tired, but if Gus would help with supervising the children, cleaning the dishes, and getting ready for bed in the evenings instead of watching TV, she could take some time for a leisurely bath—instead of her usual hurried shower—and develop some loving thoughts while she relaxed in the warm water. The issue of seeing sex as something pleasurable for herself was still the hardest task for Claire.

And there was yet another issue: As mentioned earlier, when Gus did not get what he wanted he tended to hide his disappointment behind sarcastic remarks. Gaining awareness of the effects of each partner's interaction style on their relationship was the next step in the therapy process. At this point, individuals are given a rating form to assess their own interaction style—as much as they are aware of it. In addition, they also rate on another form the characteristics of their significant others as they perceive them in their interactions. A blank copy of the Interaction Style Scale (ISS) is provided in Appendix A.

Identifying Interaction Styles

Both Gus and Claire described their own interaction styles as defensive and argumentative as well as friendly and outgoing, among other characteristics. Claire also pointed to the sarcasm Gus employed at times, although she admitted that she could hold her own in that area, as already described in the previous chapter. They were surprised at how similar they were in their interaction styles. Being confronted with these characteristics, as they had rated them, helped them realize that change was extremely important and that the sooner it took place, the better, before their feelings for each other deteriorated further.

Modifying Ineffective Interaction Styles

Except for the sexual relationship, Gus had no other issues to complain about. He loved Claire as much as he ever did, but wanted more than the occasional "charity sex." Progress did not resemble a straight upward climb; there were enough dips along the way to put the outcome in doubt. For some time, for either of them not to respond in an angry or sarcastic manner to the other partner was as difficult a task as any. Repeated confrontations with the consequences of such behaviors finally facilitated the reduction—if not extinction—of their impulsive verbal responses.

When previously they had acted on their hurt feelings and the desire to hide those feelings from each other, sarcastic remarks had become the first line of defense, especially for Gus. They had had years of practice in which to perfect their biting interaction skills. What they did not realize during those years was that their behaviors did not bring about an improvement in their situation. Focusing on the partner's shortcomings kept them from observing the detrimental effects of their own behaviors.

When asked why it had been so important to them to hide their hurt feelings from each other, they were stunned by the question. Gus responded first by saying that acknowledging wounded feelings would be a sign of weakness, whereas the expression of anger could be regarded as a demand for change or better treatment. Did he observe any change or better treatment as a result of expressing his anger? Gus admitted that the only change that had occurred was a worsening of the situation.

It took many tiny steps to get to the day when Claire appeared for their session, stating that Gus had been called out of town with his job, but he wanted the therapist to know that he was happy. Therapy did not end there but—upon their request—sessions were scheduled less frequently: from monthly to bi-monthly check-up meetings. Claire and Gus wanted to avoid falling back into their old behavior patterns. With their long-standing habit of sarcastic verbal exchanges, Claire and Gus needed reminders about modification of their interaction styles.

Lisa: Redefining Goals

Returning for now to Lisa, the young woman mentioned in Chapter 2, who had received testosterone supplement treatment and reported a "change of attitude" when her interest in sex increased despite subnormal testosterone levels, we can now focus in more detail on the mechanism for her changed attitude. Lisa's challenge had been established at the beginning of treatment as wanting to increase her sexual interest. In order to meet the challenge she had to redefine her goal. In the past, Lisa complied with sex initiated by her husband because she wanted to please him. What should her new goal be? Sexual activities should be in some way exciting—or, at least, pleasing—for her. How could this be accomplished?

In earlier sessions a more basic attitude had surfaced: Lisa regarded sex to be "dirty," although she was not able to point to anything in her past that would have given her this impression. Lisa had been raised in a small southern town and further explorations revealed that her parents never talked about sex—at least not to their children. The connection between silence and dirt made sense to Lisa as she had fabricated it in her own mind. Lisa's therapist had remembered the earlier struggle with the notion of sex being dirty and knew it needed further exploration.

Attempts to convince Lisa that there was nothing dirty about sex carried the risk of building up resistance in Lisa's mind. Yet work needed to be done to prevent Lisa from engaging in sexual activities while she was still holding the belief. Without change in her underlying beliefs, sexual intercourse would only have reinforced the notion of sex being dirty. Even feeling as she did, Lisa would have dutifully complied again with her husband's wishes. This is what women do well; as discussed in Chapter 5, they are experts in complying with the wishes of others.

Lisa was astonished to hear her therapist ask how, in her mind, sex could be made inviting. Her answer came fast and she seemed surprised by it: Elegant! Glamorous! What would keep Lisa from designing her role and environment in such a way that she would feel glamorous during sex? Lisa went to work on her new task.

In order to make sex inviting and worth engaging in for Lisa, she had to be willing and able to design her own role in it. If sex was appealing to her as a glamorous woman in an elegant setting, then therapy could assist in freeing her from the opinions of others—or what she thought their opinions were—and setting the stage appropriately for her own enjoyment.

Twice during the initial phase in therapy Lisa had mentioned that she should be less materialistic and strive to be more spiritual instead. Of course, increasing one's level of spirituality may be a healthy goal for many; however, Lisa's statement of being materialistic had the ring of criticism to it—criticism that most likely originated not from within but from someone in her environment. Making a connection between "materialistic" on the one hand and "glamorous" and "elegant" on the other provides information about a struggle concerning her wishes and the opinions of others. The conflict Lisa experienced was that as an interior decorator she and her friend and business partner worked hard to provide elegance and glamour for their clients, but she felt guilty applying her talents to her own environment. For Lisa the issue was more than having sex with her husband, the man she loved, and more than her testosterone level; it was about giving herself the freedom to arrange her world in such a way that she felt special and important in it.

In summary, before Lisa could start mapping out an approach to achieving her goal a few previously hidden obstacles had to be removed. Once that had been accomplished, she worked on designing her new sexual identity. Lisa's husband was delighted with her new approach to sex.

General Recommendations for Working on Desire Issues

In general, when treating low sexual desire, therapists encourage clients to engage in erotic responses through self-stimulation and the use of arousing fantasies. Relaxation exercises along with appropriate information gathering are important for the reduction of anxiety. Spending time as a couple in sensate focus exercises can be beneficial for lowering anxiety levels. Open and meaningful communication is of paramount importance for building emotional and physical intimacy and enhancing sexual experiences. It takes skill to initiate desired sexual activity successfully and it takes skill to refuse undesired sexual activity in a manner that does not seem complaining or accusatory.

Jim and Judy: The Contagious Effect of Moods on Sexual Desire

Judy was following the suggestion of a close friend when she called a therapist for an appointment. She sounded hesitant over the phone and admitted to being scared because she had never thought of being involved in therapy. She arrived early for her appointment and apologized three times within the first 10 minutes for things she had no responsibility for. When asked what she wanted to talk about she started to cry. While tears were rolling down her cheeks she stammered, "I was afraid that you would ask me that and I have no answer. I don't know why I am here but my friend insisted that I come." The therapist inquired gently whether there had been any changes in her life recently, to which she answered, "the only change has been that life seems so dreary lately."

It was a beginning and the therapist asked Judy to elaborate on her answer. As it turned out, Judy was less than 2 years into her current marriage and—as she stated—she should be happy because she got to marry the man she loved. He was wonderful; they had found a suitable house that they turned into a comfortable home. They were both healthy and could live on their two salaries without worry. But Judy had ceased to be her usual perky self. Why wasn't she happy? When the therapist inquired about sexual satisfaction in the marriage Judy brushed it off with, "Oh, that's okay."

The therapist gently probed about how her days went and Judy reported that her job—although safe and well-paid—was dull and unexciting. Most of her coworkers seemed depressed or bitter and resentful. "After spending the whole day in that atmosphere, I am down in the dumps myself when I come home. And what is worse, Jim, my husband, is facing a similar situation at his workplace. He works so hard among people who just hang around and do next to nothing. Yet they get promotions that should be given to him," Judy explained. "How are you able to cheer each other up?" asked the therapist. "That's just it, we are dragging each other down!" Judy replied, "And a lot of it is probably my fault. Why did I say our sex life is okay? It isn't, really."

The story that unfolded in that first session was that both spouses, unhappy in their work situation, brought the unhappiness home, and instead of focusing on the fact that they were together and away from work, they continued to drown themselves in the dreariness of their jobs by complaining about it and rehashing unpleasant events. Judy especially got so down that she was not in the mood for sex even though Jim tried to initiate it frequently—at least until recently. Now his attempts seem less frequent and less determined, leaving Judy with the nagging feeling that she has become less desirable.

Both Judy and Jim had been married before. Judy and her previous husband had tried hard to become parents, but even the expensive fertility treatments they underwent had been unsuccessful. Judy thinks she could have resigned herself to a life without children but her husband was deeply disappointed; he wanted to raise sons to continue with the family business. Of course, it did not take long before Judy blamed herself for her husband's disappointment. The marriage deteriorated to the point of divorce. Within a year after the divorce Judy's ex-husband married Judy's younger sister Kim and when the news of Kim's pregnancy was announced within the family, Judy received another blow to her already bruised self-esteem. Judy took a job in another state; she did not want to be a constant witness to her ex-husband's new family life.

Jim's previous marriage had also ended in divorce. After his son and daughter had graduated from college, Jim's wife announced that she wanted to be free to pursue a life and career of her own. After the children were gone Jim and his former wife realized that their relationship had devolved—they were more like roommates or friendly acquaintances. Their divorce was amicable and they remained on friendly terms where their children's issues were concerned.

When Judy and Jim met it became soon apparent that Jim adored Judy's warm, caring, lively, and fun-loving personality. Judy felt totally accepted and safe in Jim's adoration. It was a significant change for her from the dynamics in her first marriage. Their lovemaking was passionate and wonderful. Judy acquired a wardrobe of seductive lingerie. It seemed that their love and passion would go on indefinitely. Their values and beliefs were compatible, and the issue of children was immaterial in this marriage because Jim had no wishes to raise another family.

In her therapy session Judy came to realize that not only had their work-related disappointment been contagious between them, she had actually slowly curtailed Jim's initiation of sexual activities. In the mornings, when they left for work, she gave Jim encouraging sexual hints, but by the time they returned home, the depressing work atmosphere had taken its toll and she did not consider romantic or sexual activities. Jim, remembering the morning's verbal interchange, tried to get her involved in lovemaking, but more often than not she was not in the mood for it. When she looked back on this development, Judy was not surprised that Jim's efforts had become less ardent. She decided she needed reminders during the day to give some thought to sex and to retrieve her lingerie from the bottom of her drawer.

The lesson to be learned from this story is how easy it is to slip into a self-defeating routine and how vulnerable to extinction once-vibrant sexual passions can become in a generally depressing atmosphere. It takes awareness, time, energy, and caring to grow the fragile seeds of love and passion. Of course, one could make a case for Judy's predisposition toward low self-esteem, as she experienced it in her previous marriage and it might have been instrumental in the development of the dynamics in her current marriage. Yes, when Jim's efforts at sexual activity diminished in intensity, she assumed that he did not find her as attractive anymore. Thus, her thoughts did rather quickly turn into a negative direction—another factor she needed to become aware of. In light of her strong tendency toward self-blame, it would be beneficial for her to challenge those self-defeating cognitive paths by questioning their basis in reality.

Although Judy experienced some difficulty in the beginning of therapy with verbalizing her reasons for seeking help, it did not take her long to recognize her challenge—to revive her sexual interest, and to develop options, such as thinking more about sex and retrieving her sexy lingerie.

Another point of interest is why Jim did not clearly communicate his disappointment in Judy's responses to his sexual advances. Was he afraid to appear too demanding or might he have been scared of having to accept a verbal confirmation of Judy's rejecting behavior? Both Jim and Judy might want to explore how their interaction styles led to situations like the one that brought Judy into therapy.

The fact that his talents were apparently unappreciated in his work situation might have resulted in a lowering of Jim's individual sense of self-worth, which, in turn, could have been expected to have a profound effect on his sexuality. Because Jim was not present in the sessions, these questions remain unanswered (they may resurface later). It would also be beneficial if both Judy and Jim would search for either more interesting jobs or for ways to supplement their jobs with other stimulating work-related activities that could steer them into different career paths.

In the application of this treatment model, awareness of inefficient social skills or ineffective interaction styles that lead to undesirable consequences in the couple's interactions would be identified as factors in the challenge part and as possible choices in the options part of the model. When exploring various options that hopefully will lead to the desired goals, interaction styles again will be identified and modified to be included into behavior practices for purposeful and goal-directed behaviors. These processes are part of cognitive-behavioral approaches and can be applied in different settings, such as individual, conjoint, group, and single-sided relationship therapy; the basic underlying concepts remain the same in all settings.

Application to Group Process

Both the Hartman and Fithian and the Arentewicz and Schmidt sex therapy approaches discussed earlier have expanded their treatment modalities to include groups, in particular, couples groups. Patients may feel less uneasy with couples-group therapy if their involvement happens to be in a location away from their hometowns, so that they would not have to face the risk of running into group members after having disclosed so much personal material. Also, to make the process efficient, it is beneficial to establish homogeneous groups in terms of the presenting symptoms.

Groups homogeneous in gender as well as in symptom presentation, such as therapy groups for women suffering from vaginismus (Gehring & Chan, 2001) or hypoactive sexual desire (Trudel et al., 2001) have demonstrated successful outcomes; and the climate often found in gender-specific groups may contribute to the overall success. Although homogeneity is beneficial generally, here it is less important to focus on homogeneity of symptoms than it is in couples groups. Participants with a variety of complaints can learn from each other in the application of theoretical and practical foundations to a range of problems, as these principles can be generalized to many life areas. Attitudes and emotional reactions to various issues are usually more alike in gender-homogeneous groups than in mixed-gender groups, and members' understanding is facilitated in same-sex groups.

Application of the Model in Group Settings

In groups, the process is especially facilitated during the challenge and option phases as group members participate actively and learn from each other.

The Challenging Phase in a Group Setting

Discussing the topic of sexual desire in a group setting brought various responses from the female participants (Maass, 2002). The therapist, remembering that one of the members had previously mentioned having little interest in sexual activities, inquired if this was a recent occurrence. Jody, a group member, replied that with her husband it had been a problem for some years. She would just reluctantly give in to having sex after he had complained for several weeks. She added that at the beginning of a relationship the excitement about being with this new person would bring Jody heightened sexual interest. She admired intelligent men and wanted to please them. When they acknowledged her, Jody felt a thrill, not unlike sexual excitement.

Actually, Jody considered herself more a romantic than a sexual being, and she lost interest when the romance ended as it had in her marriage. With the arrival of children, sexual interest was replaced by general exhaustion and sex itself became a chore.

Betty, a somewhat older, divorced woman in the group, agreed with Jody that after a full day's work she did not have much energy left for sex. But Betty considered sex to be an obligation of the marriage that she had to fulfill and she had never turned her husband down—even if she did not enjoy it at the time. This made her all the more bitter when her husband became interested in a recently widowed female member of their church congregation. "He must have found the widow more exciting than me. I worked hard and hardly spent any money on myself. Every penny was spent on our sons and my husband's business; but the widow gets what she wants from him," Betty added angrily.

Inge, another group member, a beautiful, divorced and remarried woman, compared her own sexuality within her two marriages. In her first marriage sex was not exciting. She and her husband had been raised in very modest families and they never experimented sexually. In her second marriage she enjoyed her body and the pleasure it gave her husband. Inge became excited observing her husband's desire for her.

Anita, another group member, surprised the others when she likened sex to a job, but an enjoyable one. She admitted that she needed to be rested to enjoy sex. She liked to dress up in special clothes and to wear perfume, making herself as beautiful as she could. As in Inge's experience, her arousal increased with the man's increased desire for her. Anita added that Jody apparently had made a transition from romantic lover to primarily being a mother.

Jody replied angrily that this was not a matter of choice once there were children to take care of. After all, the children need monitoring and assistance, as they cannot live independently. The therapist agreed with Jody that taking care of children is a big responsibility, and that motherhood makes the woman's role very complex because it incorporates so many aspects and responsibilities. Anita's comment was made in the context of balancing these different aspects and responsibilities rather than completely abandoning one or the other of them.

This particular interaction took place during a session in the challenge phase of the group experience. Her sexual attitude was Jody's challenge. The therapist rephrased Jody's current challenge as the requirement of sexual activity in her marriage. What were the options available to her, assuming that she did not want to leave the marriage? Jody could continue to act on her negative attitudes and become cognizant of the possibility that her husband might embark upon extra-marital affairs or that the marriage might eventually dissolve.

Another option might be to discuss her feelings with her husband and agree to his seeking sexual satisfaction outside the marriage. Jody did not entertain this option. Or she could search within herself for what would improve her enjoyment of sex with her husband. In other words (similar to the situation with Lisa described in Chapters 2 and 9), what would have to happen in order for her to enjoy sexual activities? If she longed for more excitement, could she possibly provide it herself? And how?

Anita's statements were encouraging here with regard to the exploration of options. If Jody needed more time for herself to rest and prepare mentally and physically for enjoying sex, how could she schedule her activities to make that time available? For instance, what chores could her husband take on, and how could she ask him to take those chores on without creating resentment?

"Why should I have to worry about how to communicate my needs to my husband; shouldn't he know what he needs to do to help me? Not only am I doing all the chores, now I am the one who has to say things the right way?" Jody might ask. The answer would be that the goal has to be set for Jody, the woman, not the man; it is her goal. If the woman wants to improve her marriage or her sexual relationship with her husband, it is (or should be) for her own happiness mainly. Implicit in the challenge is the requirement that the woman knows herself and the boundaries she needs to establish for her happiness.

It is important to point out here that it is Jody's decision whether she wants to keep the sexual aspects of her marriage active and make those experiences enjoyable for herself. Exploration of the challenge may well include the likelihood of her husband staying in or leaving the marriage in the absence of an improved sexual relationship. It would not be therapeutic to emphasize that sex is a part of marriage and that Jody needs to participate in it if she wants to stay married. She has probably heard that already. In addition, Betty's statements indicated that this might not be a workable solution. The main thrust of Jody's work at this point is to explore what she wants and what she is willing to do to get what she wants.

After finding out what is really important to her, she can start exploring options and negotiating conditions. For instance, if Jody chose not to participate at all in sexual activities with her husband, the decision about the future of the marriage would probably be mainly in her husband's hands, and Jody would not need to do further work, except perhaps to prepare herself for a life on her own.

If, however, Jody wanted to continue with her marriage and become sexually responsive again to her husband, she would do well to explore what would put her into a romantic or erotic mood. This could consist of a small surprise, such as flowers or candy, from her husband, reading erotic literature, fantasizing about previous lovemaking, listening to romantic music—among many other things. Once she determined the tools to prepare her mood, Jody could go about installing them into her daily life.

Although the other group members faced different challenges at this time in the group's development, their expressed opinions, experiences, and attitudes helped to broaden the challenging and goal-setting parts of Jody's situation. An additional lesson could be found in Betty's situation. Perhaps at times her unenthusiastic compliance with her husband's sexual needs revealed her underlying lack of desire for participating in it. Like Gus, discussed earlier, Betty's husband might have felt unappreciated because of the "charity" sex that he received from Betty. Including sex, she had put her own wishes last, which resulted in a less than joyful atmosphere between the spouses and within the family. A look at Betty's interaction style at the time could have been helpful.

Single-Sided Relationship Therapy

Traditionally, family and marriage therapy is conducted within conjoint sessions and there are many benefits to this arrangement. However, there may be situations when conjoint sessions are impossible perhaps because one of the partners refuses to participate, or one of the partners is physically not available—perhaps because of military service or due to imprisonment.

There are also situations where conjoint sessions are ill-advised: e.g., if they provide one of the spouses with material for continuing disputes at home. The controlling spouse may use material from the conjoint session as ammunition for blaming the other or may attempt to appoint him- or herself to act as co-therapist. Another aspect of conjoint sessions is the risk of diffusion of responsibility. With both partners present, neither might feel the need to assume responsibility for change; instead, each might wait for the other to do so. A viable alternative in cases like those described above would be to use a single-sided relationship therapy model (Maass, 2005).

The potential for clients' increased control and independence becomes apparent when working with single parents (Maass & Neely, 2000). These clients are required to handle several different relationship adjustments almost simultaneously; there are relationships with ex-spouses, parents, parents-in-law, siblings-in-law, children, and possibly new romantic attachments to consider. It would be unrealistic to expect all involved to participate in therapy with the single-parent client. Recognizing this fact makes it possible to generalize the skills involved in the work with single parents to other relationship constellations within the general population.

How does single-sided relationship therapy differ from regular individual therapy? As would be expected, the setting is similar to that of individual therapy in that the therapist works with one client at the time. The main difference is the focus of the work. Whereas in individual therapy the client may reveal several issues dealing with a range of circumstances in her life, the work in single-sided relationship therapy—based on the client's wishes—is focused on the client's relationship with a particular person. As the focus is narrowed to the relationship and the other person in that relationship, it also becomes more intense in the application of the whole process.

Reactions and responses of the other person are anticipated and considered as if the other person were present in the session. Knowing the interaction style of the other allows the client to evaluate the estimated responses of the absent person and helps the client formulate his or her next step. She may even want to rehearse her verbalizations and behavior again, after considering the possible responses from the partner. Of course, there are areas of overlap between the two approaches.

Applied Single-Sided Relationship Therapy to Sexual Desire Issues

In the experience of many practitioners, requests for marriage or family therapy are frequently initiated by women. Although it does happen from time to time, it is rare that a man makes the first call for an appointment. Why is the woman so often the one who initiates therapy? Is it because she has more time to make the call or she knows the family's schedule? Is it because she assumes the responsibility for the emotional quality of the relationship?

Usually she is the one willing to admit that she hurts, and she hopes that with the help of the therapist her husband or her children will understand how they are hurting her and they will somehow be made to change. Spouses who have heard the complaints before will be armed with a negative attitude at the beginning of therapy. They will be ready to defend their positions and point out the unreasonableness in the other's requests.

In the ideal case of marriage or sex therapy, all involved have a common goal—improvement of the situation they are currently in. However, there are couples who overtly profess to have a common goal while covertly one of the spouses wants the other to change and the other resists the change, instead expecting things to improve without actually doing anything different. This scenario includes two actors with different—perhaps even opposing—goals, each proceeding in his or her unique problem-solving style. In still other cases, the presenting problem may be the element that keeps the unit together in more-or-less haphazard ways, and low desire may function in maintaining the balance.

Norma: Doing It by Herself

Norma, a married mother of four children, had made the phone call to schedule an appointment for herself and her husband. When they arrived for their initial session, Norma spoke first, introducing herself and then Ron as a good, hard-working husband, who provided well for the family. Norma swallowed hard and then blurted out, "Our biggest problem is that I don't want as much sex as Ron does." Her high-pitched voice betrayed the anxiety she felt at the time.

With that one sentence, Norma had assumed the blame for any of the difficulties that may have existed in their marriage, and this was not lost on Ron, who confirmed, "She never wants sex; she is either too tired or doesn't feel good, or is worried about the children waking up. I am the one who locks our bedroom door at night. I am also the one who brings the children over to their grandparents' house. But it makes her feel obligated, she says, that she now has to have sex—no matter how she really feels." Ron turned to the therapist. "See, no matter what I do, it is not enough. How would you feel if your spouse never wanted to have sex with you?" Ron attempted both to challenge the therapist and at the same time to align himself with the therapist. It was easy to see that Ron was used to establishing control in situations he was involved in.

Many therapists schedule individual sessions for the spouses to facilitate the communication of their concerns without being afraid that the other spouse will be critical, will misunderstand, or feel hurt. For Norma and Ron, individual sessions were indicated as soon as possible. Norma was the first one to be seen individually. She reported how after the session ended Ron had lectured her about her shortcomings. He tried to reinterpret some of the therapist's statements so that they agreed with his own position. It came down to this: all Norma had to do was change her attitude about his sexual needs and her responsibility. They would not need to see a therapist for that.

When it was time for Ron's individual session, Norma called and apologized that Ron would not be able to keep the appointment. She was willing to come instead to avoid wasting the therapist's time. The therapist explored options with Norma: She could wait until her husband was able to participate in conjoint sessions and then hope to work out some of their difficulties. Or she could forget about therapy and trying to change altogether. Or she could work individually on improving the relationship or her own feelings.

The speed with which Norma answered indicated that she had already given some thought to the situation, "I think, for the time being I would like to come and see you by myself. After the first session I realized that it would not be easy for me to address the reasons for my lack of interest in sex with my husband present. It is not just one or two little things that make me not want to have sex."

Acknowledging Norma's statement, the therapist started to address the challenging situation in more concrete terms. Based on Ron's statements during and after the initial session and Norma's own expectations, what would be the challenge in the therapy process? Answer: To improve their sexual relationship. What was necessary to accomplish that? Norma replied that Ron saw the need for Norma to change her attitude and to be willingly and enthusiastically available for sexual activities. If that was Ron's goal, what strategy had he employed so far to reach his goal?

Norma admitted that he had at times taken the responsibility of bringing the children to his parents, but mostly he had been complaining about Norma's lack of enthusiasm. Ron's behavior did not indicate that he would be willing to change his behavior or give up something without getting something in return. He saw himself already as giving more than he was getting.

What would be Norma's goal in therapy? Answer: To improve her level of sexual desire. How would she go about reaching her goal? Norma had no immediate answer. What were the underlying reasons for her lack of sexual desire? When she had identified what kept her from wanting to be physically and emotionally intimate with the man she was married to, she could assume the responsibility for changes she could make in herself which in turn could be expected to bring about some changes in Ron's attitudes and behavior. The therapist started to outline the process to Norma.

After identification of the underlying reasons, what strategies might work best for Norma? The answer to this question will come out of a detailed exploration of behavioral options available to her. It is important to make sure that the options she might choose are congruent with her values and beliefs; otherwise she will not be successful with her new behaviors.

During the action phase of the therapy process Norma would devote her energies to practicing her behavioral strategies and to observing the results. At this point Norma remarked again that for her it would be easier to discuss behavioral strategies and their application with the therapist in individual sessions because she would feel awkward in disclosing these aspects in conjoint sessions before practicing them because Ron might be critical of her attempts.

For the time being, Norma seemed to prefer the single-sided approach to therapy. The therapist informed Norma that it would take a lot of work, and sometimes it might be discouraging to think that she was the primary person doing the work. She might even think that there was something wrong with her. On the other hand, exploring what she wanted and thinking about ways how to get it would help her to feel more confident in herself. What had started out as conjoint therapy for the time being turned into single-sided relationship therapy.

It was not difficult to see that Norma felt she carried the major burden of the sexual problem. As she had stated at the beginning of the first visit, she acknowledged herself to be the cause of the problem. Ron had eagerly agreed with her. This was typical of many of their interactions.

How had the emotional atmosphere been early in their relationship, when they were dating? the therapist inquired. Norma replied that she had felt safe with Ron; he was so knowledgeable and she had looked up to him. He seemed more patient then and explained things to her. She added that he seemed to enjoy telling her about things she did not know. What had attracted her to him sexually at the beginning? Norma thought for a moment before replying as tears filled her eyes,

"The way he smiled at me. It was a warm, approving smile, which made me feel special. His hands felt good too when he touched me, so strong but gentle."

"What, would you say, Ron liked about you when you were dating?" The therapist asked. "He used to say that he liked the way I listened to him; it gave him the impression that I gave him my undivided attention and that he was important to me." Norma responded.

The therapist followed with a question: If Norma had to pinpoint a time when their emotional atmosphere seemed to have changed, when would that have been? Again, Norma had to think for a moment but remembered that after the birth of their second child things slowly changed. There seemed to be less time for her and Ron just to be by themselves and usually she seemed to be so tired in the evenings. Norma remembered that one evening after their third child was about a year old Ron was telling her about an article he had been reading in the paper that caught his attention. Unfortunately, Norma fell asleep as Ron talked. He made a joke about it the next day, but he did not laugh. Since then Ron had become more critical of her.

Could it be that in addition to the reduced frequency of sex due to Norma's exhaustion, Ron had missed the attention and adoration he had received from Norma at the beginning of their relationship? If so, he might have been hiding his disappointment and hurt feelings behind criticizing Norma, perhaps in a similar way as Gus (who had been hiding his hurt feelings behind sarcasm) did in his relationship with Claire.

Norma was asked to rate her own and Ron's interaction styles. She thought that Ron interacted with her in a criticizing—and at times—impatient and dismissing manner. What did she think were Ron's thoughts about her? "Oh, he is probably disgusted that I can't cope with our lives more efficiently. I am always behind with things. Raising four children is harder than I thought it would be." Norma sounded hopeless as she answered the question.

And how would Norma describe her own interaction style? She seemed puzzled; she had not thought about it, but then she admitted that she was defensive because she frequently felt accused. She also acknowledged feeling angry often but did not dare express it openly. Her way was to withdraw into silence when defending herself did not work. Her silent, smoldering anger also made her unapproachable, she admitted.

"So you act in a defensive way toward Ron because you think he is disgusted with your lack of coping skills, is that it?" the therapist inquired. After Norma's confirmation, the therapist followed up with Norma's earlier statement about Ron's liking it when Norma in the past had listened to him attentively. Was it really true that Ron was disgusted, or could he be disappointed at the reduced attention he received from Norma? Norma admitted that in interpreting Ron's behavior she had assumed he was disgusted. Over time, the assumption had become a belief, and the character of much of her responding behavior was based on that belief.

In interpreting others' behaviors we often fill in the gaps in our actual knowledge with assumptions. If our perception of the behavior is negative, most likely we will respond in a somewhat negative manner, which in turn would result in a less than positive reaction from the other. This reaction would reinforce our original negative perception and strengthen the belief that our perception was accurate. As we continue to act as if our beliefs are true and our perceptions are accurate, the vicious cycle goes on.

Obviously, their interaction styles were not destined to improve the situation. In order to be heard, Norma needed to challenge or explore the accuracy of her perceptions and her beliefs before formulating her response. She was diligent in exploring different approaches—always trying to anticipate Ron's likely response and paying attention to her emotional reactions to those responses. If the responses Norma anticipated from Ron made her anger increase, she needed to be aware of that and then consider trying a different approach.

How did Ron usually respond to her defensive silence? "He raises his eyebrows as he looks at me, then shakes his head and walks away, mumbling, 'Here we go again!' That makes me even more angry but also feeling very lonely." How would Norma want him to respond? "I want him to validate me. I want him to listen to me when I defend myself and to recognize that I have valid reasons to be angry." Then in a low tone of voice, she added, "Perhaps he is doing the same thing I do?" Norma added. The therapist agreed that this was likely the case, because people are so used to letting their perceptions go by unchallenged as to their correctness in reality and to forming a belief system around them that remains equally unchallenged. Similar dynamics had been operating in the cases of Claire and Gus and Judy and Jim discussed earlier.

Norma learned how she could change this cycle of misperceptions, negative feelings, and misunderstandings. It was painstaking work for Norma, but it eventually gave her a sense of control over their communication. Before working on resolutions to any of their problems, Norma and Ron had to be able to listen and talk to each other. Many steps needed to be taken—from improving their communication style to improving their sex life. For instance, Norma's statement about her valid reasons for anger needed further attention. People often ask, "Don't I have a right to be angry?" This makes it sound as if feeling anger is a privilege. In reality, however, behind the question lies the unspoken demand that the culprit should acknowledge having caused the irritation, apologize, and make restitution. It seldom works that way, though. Therefore, the person experiencing the anger might better search for more self-enhancing ways to handle the feelings and the expression of anger.

The reader may remember that Norma had stated her goal as wanting to improve her level of sexual desire, but she did not know how to do that. This is not surprising because she had never determined within herself what purpose sex served for her. Was it to enjoy the sensuous experiences that sexual activity can give? Was it to make Ron happy? Was the purpose of sex to have children? Her answer was "all of the above," but it did not ring true and she admitted that she had never thought about this in any detail. After all, sex was a natural act, serving different functions, and—above all—it should come naturally.

Norma is not alone in her beliefs; as outlined in Chapter 4, many girls and women are not encouraged during their development to contemplate seriously what sex might mean to them and what would make sex not only acceptable, but also enjoyable to them. The topic of sexual satisfaction was briefly raised in Chapter 3. The term is ambiguous because there are many different definitions of sexual satisfaction. Basically, the word *satisfaction* indicates that we like what happened or we agree with what we received. Thus, satisfaction can be obtained by different means.

Explorations, aided by a sample of lists about conditions that would likely help Norma to experience an interest in sex and how she could arrange to have those conditions become part of her life—preferably with the help of her husband—occupied another segment of her therapy. Norma learned to become aware of what she wanted, how to get it, and to determine what she was willing to do for getting it.

Because their unhappy situation had developed over a period of years and because of the fact that Ron was not participating in therapy, it was Norma's task to find opportunities to obtain Ron's assistance in the overall process. What would make it desirable for Ron to help? How could Norma plan and implement strategies that would lead Ron to participate willingly in the process of change?

Some may ask, "Why should Norma have to worry about all that; shouldn't Ron be willing to do his share to improve the relationship?" The answer is it would be nice if Ron willingly participated and Norma would be delighted if he did. It is, however, Norma's life and Norma's marriage and if she is willing to assume the full responsibility for both, she is entitled to the rewards of not only being in a happier relationship with her husband but also of feeling confident and competent within herself.

TABLE 10.1. Things That Would Make Me Interested in Having Sex

What I can do to feel desire	What my partner can do	My partner's response
1. Read erotic literature	1. Smile at me	
2. View pornography	2. Call me during the day to tell me he/she misses me	
3. Listen to romantic music	3. Leave little notes hidden for me to find telling me he/she loves me	
4. Take a leisurely bath, play with myself	4. Bring me flowers or candy	
5. Fantasize about previous lovemaking with my partner	5. Kiss me passionately	
6. Fantasize about lovemaking with someone else I know	6. Help me with chores/errands	
7. Fantasize about lovemaking with a stranger	7. Take me out for dinner or a show	
8. Use my favorite perfume, dress sexy	8. Tell me I am beautiful	
9. Have a glass of wine/beer/cocktail	9. Give me a massage	
10. Other	10. Take a shower with me	
	11. Other	

11
Learning From the Past—Thoughts for the Future

The author of the *Science* article previously mentioned in Chapter 3 (Enserink, 2005) reported that researchers have found most women's sexual complaints to be connected to self-respect, self-image, and relationship quality, which are psychological issues. Clinical psychologist Leonore Tiefer, who gave a presentation at the December meeting of the U.S. Food and Drug Administration, is quoted as calling the current pharmaceutical focus "medicalization" of female sexuality, while Irwin Goldstein of Boston University calls it "psycholization."

Tiefer (2001) calls on feminists to "scrutinize all sexual prescriptions offered for women, especially those that seem to suggest women's sexual experience would be better, more normal, or more fulfilling, if it more closely paralleled men's" (p. 84). In the second edition of her book *Sex Is Not a Natural Act,* Tiefer (2004) proposed viewing sex in social terms as a psychophysiological potential that can be developed to different levels, depending on the participants' interests and opportunities.

As discussed previously, the relevant literature contains substantiation that women desire sex less often than men (Baumeister, Catanese, & Vohs, 2001). Lauman and colleagues (1994) in their national probability-sampled data reported that 33.4% of the women reported a lack of sexual interest for several months or more, compared with 15.8% of men. Many wives would probably not miss sexual activities if they never again occurred in their lives.

Examining women's life cycles regarding sexual interest beginning in childhood and adolescence through the reproductive years, midlife, and older age, Leiblum and Sachs (2002) listed a menu of opportunities, such as cybersex, hormone treatment, medication, cosmetic and reproductive surgery, mind–body practices, and therapy, that are supposed to assist women in achieving the sexual experiences they want. But the authors cautioned that for the many women who are affected by a lack of sexual desire, getting back blood flow and lubrication (which could be restored by some of the pharmaceutical agents that are on the market now or in various stages of development) are just the tip of the iceberg. These vasodilating drugs won't do anything if a woman does not have the desire for sex. Continuing the discussion, the authors pointed out that some of the studies reported in the literature have demonstrated that even women who did not receive the experimental treatment reported an improvement in their sexual experiences. In other words, the placebo effect is still at work—if one does anything and believes in it, one's sex life may improve.

Does Low Sexual Interest Become a Dysfunction in the Process of Medicalization?

Individuals tend to resent being labeled with a "disorder" just because they have little or no interest in sex. "If someone does not like to eat broccoli, is that a disorder?" one woman asked. Professionals have expressed "a very real and valid concern that the treatment of sexual complaints and sexuality in general could potentially become medicalized, much like the treatment of premature ejaculation" (Berman & Berman, 2000, p. 17). But as pharmaceutical companies require sex therapists to be at the treatment sites for their clinical trials for sexual dysfunction, they seem to have realized that drugs are not the sole answer for women who fail to become sexually interested.

Answers From a Biopsychosocial Perspective

To examine how levels of sexual desire are associated with various biopsychosocial factors was the purpose of the American Association of Retired Persons' (AARP) *Modern Maturity* Sexuality Survey, a mail survey completed by 1,384 women and men aged 45 and older. Measures for level of sexual desire included information on the frequency of sexual desire as expressed in thoughts, fantasies, or erotic dreams. The results showed that among women, age, high blood pressure, prescription medications, negative attitudes toward sexuality, absence of a sexual partner, and low household income were correlated with low sexual desire (DeLamater & Sill, 2005).

For the men in the sample, age, high blood pressure, enlarged prostate, anticoagulants and medications for hypertension, absence of a sexual partner, negative attitude toward sexual activity, and low income were all negatively correlated with reported sexual desire.

The results showed that although sexual desire decreases as women and men age, it does not decrease as fast as popular belief dictates. In this study, it is not until age 75 or older that the majority of women and almost a majority of men reported a low level of sexual desire. And significantly, except for age, the effects of attitudes were larger than the effects of any other predictor included in the analyses.

The newest AARP study conducted in 2004 surveyed 1,682 adults, aged 45 and older, about their sexual attitudes and quality of life (Jacoby, 2005). This study included the viewpoints of three-quarters of the 78 million baby-boomers as well as individuals in their 60s, 70s, 80s, and older. According to the current report, the proportion of men who have used potency-enhancing medicines has doubled since the 1999 study.

Additionally, it was reported that the men's increased use of potency-enhancing treatments is welcomed by their female partners—no matter what their age. For the 45–49-year-old group, men and women ascribed almost equal importance to sexual satisfaction, but by age 60, only 27% of women as contrasted with 62% of men placed a high value on a satisfying sexual relationship.

Interestingly, the article in the AARP Magazine mentions sociology professor Michael Kimmel as saying that drugs like Viagra, Cialis, and Levitra are not effective for every man, because they do not address emotional problems that may be affecting the man's sexual functioning. This is yet another indication that human sexuality, sexual desire, and sexual functioning are complex and involve more than just one aspect of an individual's life.

Lessons For the Future

The above-mentioned groups represent some of the voices speaking out about human sexual attitudes and function, and in particular, women's sexuality. What can we learn from them for the future? For one thing, sexuality and sexual attitudes are not confined to one particular field of research and exploration. Answers are not found solely in the fields of medicine, physiology, or pharmacology. Psychology, sociology, philosophy, religion, and other disciplines contain parts of the puzzle—and parts of the answers.

The Unrealistic Trust in the Healing Powers of Time

Although folk-myths want us to believe that "time heals all wounds," this does not apply automatically to troubled intimate relationships. As is often the case with marital therapy, if spouses seek professional help, it is usually late in the problematic situation; the scenario with sex therapy is similar. Much pain and resentment have accumulated in one or both partners because they feel rejected, neglected, or taken for granted—or even taken advantage of. The longer the partners have been together, the more likely it is that opportunities for miscommunication and misunderstandings may have taken a toll on their mutual trust and love.

It would be a therapist's dream to work with clients when problems first start to develop, or even better, beforehand, so that difficulties can be kept from evolving. How can individuals be persuaded to pay attention to the early signs of difficulty and, instead of explaining them away, focus on their resolution? For their physical health, people have come to understand the importance of periodic check-ups with their physicians. But when the frequency and intensity of sexual activities decrease in couples, they often explain it away with such reasons as "What do you expect—we have been together for quite some time; things cool down" or "We are getting older; it's natural to slow down" or "Life has just been so hectic lately" or "I am working too hard and there is not enough energy left for sex" or "We don't seem to be in the same place at the same time." These explanations may sound logical on the surface, but they function mainly to prolong the period of slowed sexual activity without initiating change.

These explanations—or excuses—also give the impression that sexuality is a static characteristic and that sexual activities are events that occur periodically and not in a continuous fashion throughout the individual's lifespan. It is not surprising then that with the growth of personal responsibilities priorities get reassigned and sex is the one that most likely ends up at the bottom of the list, as we have seen in the stories of Rhonda and Julie in Chapter 7.

Sexuality From a Developmental Perspective

"Adolescent girls do not go to sex therapists" (Tolman, 2001, p. 205). This statement makes a direct connection to a significant part of the difficulty with women's sexual desire. Sexuality is a developmental issue. It is not something the young woman wakes up with on the morning of her wedding day. Years of female adolescent experiences and myths have shaped her attitudes and beliefs. Yet not many pay attention to this development beyond some cautionary statements like "Don't get pregnant" or "Don't pick up a disease." In fact, if a young girl does not express an interest in boys or petting activities, her parents usually feel relieved. As long as she is not engaged in sex, she is "safe," and no sexuality is often equated with good or healthy sexuality. Negative consequences are avoided by avoiding the sexual experience, not by learning from it.

Holding on to the fable that good girls want love rather than sex makes thinking about sex unnecessary. "Normal" female adolescent sexuality is thought of within the framework of romance narratives. "Sexual desire is male; it is intractable, uncontrollable, and victimizing" (Tolman, 2000, p. 70). Failing to provide meaningful role models about the experience and handling of passionate sexual feelings leaves young women insufficiently prepared to face adult reality.

For different reasons, young girls or women do not spend much time contemplating sexuality. They may focus on love rather than on sex, as discussed earlier, or they may expect sexual activity to "fall into place" once they are engaging in it because they think of it as—contrary to Leonore Tiefer's notion—a natural aspect of the life they are going to experience in an intimate relationship. And often the excitement of the newness of such a relationship helps things to progress more ore less smoothly—at least in the beginning.

The belief that sex is a natural function is exactly what sex therapist David Schnarch (1997) warned about. In his opinion, the "'naturalized' view of sex is not so liberating because it pressures people to have sexual desire and sexual response, and makes worrying about sexual performance seem inappropriate" (p. 129). Comparing sexual desire to a kind of natural hunger masks its complexity and leaves people believing that they are defective if they don't experience the sexual "hunger pangs."

Clinical psychologist Mary Pipher (1994) wrote that in the 1990s in America young girls faced conflicting sexual issues. One of the issues was to learn about and to define their own sexuality, i.e., learning about sex and making choices. But another issue revolved around the danger of sexual victimization. Because of the myths and many of the double messages inherent in our culture, young boys and girls develop different attitudes about sex. There are no clearly defined rules about sexuality.

If those issues collided to make decisions about sexuality and sexual activities difficult for young girls in the 1990s, how is it different for young girls in the new millennium? Most likely, it isn't much different. The discussion of this issue in Chapter 4 does not indicate a significant change in the sexual dilemma facing young girls today.

In an informal discussion about their first sexual experiences, when they lost or gave up their virginity, about half of the young women in a college course on human sexuality admitted that it had been "awful" or "meaningless;" only a few remembered it as a good experience. Many did not know what to expect, and none of them had developed any criteria defining a situation or person with whom to have their first sexual intercourse. Some continued dating their boyfriends afterward and eventually became pregnant, while others felt abandoned and abused.

When asked what would they do differently in retrospect, many replied that they would have liked to have made the decision where to have sex rather than have the boy determine it. However, they added, that would have seemed inappropriate at the time. Why? They gave several reasons: By deciding where to have sex, the girl would make herself seem too eager and the boy would not respect her. Or, it is the boy's responsibility to determine time and place; that means he cares for her. Those were the thoughts the young women reported having had at the time of their first sexual encounter. Not all of them were still convinced that it was the best approach for them.

One obvious danger in this scenario is that the girls gave up control over what might happen to them. If they decided to change their mind and not go through with intercourse, the setting arranged by the boy may have rendered the girls helpless and unable to act on the possibility of changing their mind. At this point in the discussion two of the young women admitted that their first intercourse had actually amounted to a date rape.

Even if a young girl is receptive to a young man's ardent attempts either because she is curious about sex or does not want to hurt his feelings or does not dare say no to sexual intercourse, nobody is much concerned if she did not enjoy the experience. Without sensitive guidance about sexuality, she may do more of the same without enjoying it or she may turn away completely from sex until she becomes seriously involved in it either through marriage or cohabitation, neither one of which guarantees much better experiences.

A young woman who becomes involved in a serious relationship may know very little about what it takes to experience sexual desire or arousal. She may believe that all it takes is for her partner to push the right "buttons" on her body and sometimes that seems to work. What she often does not know is that responding to "button-pushing" might eventually turn out to be just one more undesirable act in a long list of a day's activities. Sexual activity in most married or cohabiting couples is restricted to the evenings—the end of long days. This in itself can be considered a statement about the priority of sex; as mentioned earlier, it occupies the bottom of a long list of activities.

   If the young woman has not experimented with her own sensuality, she will not know what and how long it will take for her to get into a romantic mood or to prepare herself for sex because she has not explored these aspects when she had the time available. Now, in the middle of the demands of a hectic lifestyle, there may be no time for such experimentation.

Gender Differences in Developmental Tasks

If we consider sexuality from a developmental perspective, we can also understand and accommodate the notion of differences in the developmental task between males and females. Just because males feel sexual desire faster and more frequently, that does not mean it should be the norm for females as well. Once we are able and willing to accept the idea that the internal sexuality process in females is different from that of males, we can work on a resolution that will accommodate both sexes. But as long as we deny gender-based differences, we close the door to further knowledge.

   At the same time, if we acknowledge a difference but ascribe the word *dysfunction* to the different condition, we end up searching for a "cure" more than for knowledge and understanding, while at the same time running the risk of alienating those who experience the "different condition."

The "Normal" Frequency of Sex

In a recent discussion about sexuality among college students, the focus turned to the "normal" frequency of sexual intercourse. Of course, there is no one correct answer that applies to everybody. One young female student stated that sexual activities between her and her partner had decreased in frequency lately. They were both busy with their studies and their jobs; their schedules did not accommodate much free time for sex. As she explained the situation, she tried to make the case for a "quality over quantity" arrangement.

   Her argument sounded a bit hollow and reminiscent of the excuses listed earlier in this chapter. In the area of lovemaking and intimacy, a reduction in frequency often also brings about a reduction in quality. Longer periods of time between lovemaking events can introduce awkwardness between the partners, which may take away from the natural playfulness that exists as part of true intimacy between two partners who are familiar with each other's bodies and responses. Spontaneity is best cultivated in circumstances of familiarity.

   At the next class meeting the young woman mentioned that she had brought up the class discussion to her partner. Both had reconsidered their situation and decided that they did not want to slide into a neglectful love life. They wanted to guard their intimacy carefully and therefore they decided to give top priority to their sex life. Even if they could not afford to spend whole afternoons in bed playing, they needed to make the time for frequent meaningful connections with each other. How long will they remember their resolution?

The Importance of Determining the Purpose of Sex

One step in effecting change would be to encourage young girls (and women) to define for themselves what the goal or purpose of sex should be. If a woman determines the purpose of sex to be procreation, then after the conception and birth of the desired number of children there would not be a purpose for further sexual activities. Another part of this question would be, Does the woman want the children for herself mainly or for her husband? Most would say for both. However, that is not always true. There are situations where the husband would prefer fewer or even no children but agrees to go along with his wife's wishes for more children. Recall the case history of Lynn (Chapter 7), whose husband would have preferred a childless marriage and who after fathering one child felt incapable of raising another. Lynn, however, felt deprived of having a second child due to her husband's illness and built up a long-standing resentment.

If procreation is the main reason for engaging in sex, should the woman communicate that clearly to her partner before marriage? We can think of many situations where husbands continue to have expectations for sexual activity after the desired number of offspring has been delivered. Without a clear understanding of the woman's plans and intentions, husbands in this situation might feel betrayed and tend to regard themselves as "sperm donors" rather than as lovers.

Another reason for the woman to engage in sexual activity might be to please her partner. And here again, there are two aspects to consider. If sex is strictly for the partner's pleasure, there is the risk that the woman will get tired of giving unless she receives something equally valuable in return, which is reminiscent of aspects of exchange theory discussed in earlier chapters. On the other hand, if the woman firmly believes that pleasing a husband is part of being a good wife and it is important for her own self-esteem and her own identity to be a good wife, then she will engage in sex for herself and thus will be less likely to resent it over time.

Of course, if the woman's goal for sexual activity is her own pleasure, that would be the best scenario. After finding out what she likes, she will be inclined to take on responsibility for getting what she wants by communicating that to her partner. An awareness of her sexual attitudes and her sexual interaction style would most certainly enhance the success of her communication (see Appendix C: Sex Attitude Check, a rating scale on one's sexual interaction style). The woman who wants sex for her own pleasure knows what pleases her and what attracts her to her partner. Thus, knowing the purpose a woman bestows on sexual activity might give us an insight into the probability of whether—like many women—she will or—like some women—she will not enjoy sex.

Knowing What Turns You On

The group of young college women mentioned earlier rated partners' behaviors according to what would most likely stimulate them to experience sexual desire. At the top of the list were situations when the partner called during the day or left little notes behind, which made the women feel that the partner cared for them. The partner's smile came in second in importance, before bringing small gifts like candy or flowers.

The importance of a partner's smile was noted recently with a female client who was asked about her feelings toward her partner when he smiled at her. Tears started rolling down her cheeks immediately. "He hasn't smiled at me in a long time," she replied. "Does your husband know how important his smile is to you?" asked the therapist. The client shook her head, "I don't think so." "How do you think he would respond if you told him that?" was the therapist's next question. The client thought that her husband would be surprised and that he would probably like it.

These situations demonstrate that women know what they like their partners to do to make them feel loved and cared for and, generally speaking, these feelings are better predictors of sexual interest than many other variables. But do the women clearly communicate the significance of their partners' behaviors to them? Apparently not—but why not?

Another question for our college women dealt with aspects of inducing sexual desire in themselves. The most preferred type of stimulation was fantasizing about previous lovemaking with the current partner. The least preferred kind of stimulation was listed as viewing pornography. Listening to romantic music and reading erotic literature surprisingly received relatively cool endorsements, which may indicate a shift away from the long-held notion that women respond well to romantic-erotic reading or viewing materials. Taking a leisurely bath and dressing in sexy garments were placed somewhere in the middle on the list of preferred stimuli, before the use of alcohol.

The same questionnaire was given to women in the general community. Compared with the students' answers, these women added several items that their partners could do for them; and that list eventually became longer than the list of things they could do for their own increased sexual desire.

How often did the women use their preferred type of stimulation to set the stage? The women in the community at large seemed to employ those strategies more frequently than the students, whose answers ranged from "Every time" and "Seldom" (which held the two highest spots) to "As often as I remember to do it" and "Waiting for partner to set the stage." The reason unanimously given for not using their preferred pre-sex activity to stimulate their sexual interest was "Not enough time"—due to work schedule, school, and children's needs. This was yet another indication of the limiting effects of time pressures and the priorities set by the participants.

When Celia Mosher, first mentioned in Chapter 1, obtained information about women's sexual attitudes and practices with her questionnaire, most of the 44 women who responded reported positive attitudes regarding sexual activities. It may be of interest to remember that 81% of her sample had attended college or normal school and all were economically well-off (Bullough, 1994). Being "economically well-off" at that time meant that these women probably did not work outside the home and in all likelihood enjoyed the services of paid household help—quite a different situation from many of the young women we encounter today with complaints of low libido.

Does this mean that the women of earlier generations had better or easier lives? Does it mean that today's women with the opportunities and responsibilities of fulfilling careers are worse off than the women of Celia Mosher's time? Not necessarily, but the availability of increased opportunities brings with it the responsibility to make reasonable choices. The existence of increased options does not mean we can use them all. Being a full-time employee and attending school in the evenings to prepare for a law degree while having the responsibility for three or four children may sound inspiring in an autobiography of a female chief justice, but in reality, the hardships inherent in this situation would make it difficult for many of us to remain inspired for an extended period of time.

On the other hand, one of the options we do not have anymore is to return to earlier times in history. The destabilization of marriage makes a guaranteed career as a homemaker problematic. Changing commitments to marriage and economic uncertainty constitute a realistic threat to women without a profession (or inherited money). Thus, women are faced with the necessity of selecting training for an income-producing career and in addition choosing a partner with whom they can share their lives in a harmonious atmosphere. What does all that have to do with sex? some may ask. The answer—a lot: they are all interdependent aspects of today's women's lives.

The age of innocence has come to an abrupt end for many young girls—if it ever really existed. With an eye toward preparing young females for their future, shouldn't the introduction and achievement of developmental tasks for young girls include aspects of female sexuality as well as the development of morality, personality, psychological identity, and future career considerations?

Appendix A

Interaction Style Scale (ISS)

shy	1	2	3	4	3	2	1	outgoing/ expressive
avoidant	1	2	3	4	3	2	1	involved
aggressive	1	2	3	4	3	2	1	acquiescent
domineering	1	2	3	4	3	2	1	submissive
complaining	1	2	3	4	3	2	1	accommodating
accusatory	1	2	3	4	3	2	1	defensive
conciliatory	1	2	3	4	3	2	1	confrontational
empathic	1	2	3	4	3	2	1	aloof, remote
emotional	1	2	3	4	3	2	1	logical
impulsive	1	2	3	4	3	2	1	cautious
placating	1	2	3	4	3	2	1	argumentative
intimidating	1	2	3	4	3	2	1	appeasing
demanding	1	2	3	4	3	2	1	considerate
critical	1	2	3	4	3	2	1	accepting
angry	1	2	3	4	3	2	1	calm
assertive	1	2	3	4	3	2	1	timid
harsh, rough	1	2	3	4	3	2	1	gentle
hostile	1	2	3	4	3	2	1	friendly
active	1	2	3	4	3	2	1	passive
controlling	1	2	3	4	3	2	1	laid back
compulsive	1	2	3	4	3	2	1	spontaneous
sarcastic	1	2	3	4	3	2	1	respectful

Please rate each of the personality characteristics above by circling first the word for it and then assigning a level of significance to it by circling a number from 1 to 4,with 4 being the strongest level of the characteristic that you consider the person (or you) demonstrates.

Appendix B

Recommendations

The following questions and suggestions are offered to those individuals who want to increase their awareness about their own needs, wishes, and preferences and want to make use of this awareness in planning their actions. These items do not take the place of structured exercises that may be found in other materials; they are simply suggestions to be followed as preferred.

To arrive at a realistic estimate of what it takes to lead the life one wants to enjoy, it would be beneficial for the individual woman to ask herself the following questions:

(Answers to questions 4, 5, and 6 in combination with question 2 will provide an estimate of how much time the individual woman has left over to think about sexual activities.)

1. What do I see as my purpose for engaging in sex?
    (a) procreation (b) to please my partner (c) to please myself (d) a+b+c
2. If procreation is the main purpose, how many children do I want to raise?
    (a) one (b) two (c) three (d) more than three
3. How important is career development to me?
    (a) very important (b) mildly important (c) not important at all
4. How much time (outside regular working hours) do I need/want to devote to achieve/maintain my career goals? (answer according to daily or weekly basis)
    (a) none (b) 1–2 hours/day/week (c) 3–5 hours/day/week
5. How much time do I need/want for resting, doing things for myself, being with friends, etc., (outside of sleep) to feel good and energized?
    (a) 2 hours/day/week (b) >2 hours/day/week (c) 3–5 hours/day/week
6. How much time do I need to prepare myself mentally, emotionally, and physically to enjoy sexual activities with my partner (for each event)?
    (a) 0 (b) 1–2 hours (c) 3+ hours (d) whole day

7. Which type of preparation for sexual desire works best for me?
   (a) reading erotica (b) listen to music (c) relaxing/fantasizing (d) self-pleasure (e) other—explore your own ideas, find something that works for you and that you enjoy; everybody has different wishes and preferences
8. What things can my partner do to help me get into the mood for sex?
   (a) I have a whole list (b) I can't think of any (c) I am afraid to ask (d) He should know

If you checked answer (c), what might be the reason for being afraid to ask?

If your answer is (d), does that mean you have clearly communicated what you want or should your partner be able to read your mind? When it comes to what you want, nothing should be left to chance. Your wishes are important!

Communication: It is important that your wishes as well as your dislikes are being understood accurately. When you rate your habits of communicating on the Interaction Style Scale, what are the most striking characteristics? Do you approve of them in yourself or do you detect a slight need for modification?

How would you rate your partner's interaction style? Do your interaction styles complement each other or do they introduce friction? What could be changed?

Appendix C

Sex Attitude Check

What is the overall sexual scenario with your partner—granting your partner's wishes or giving in to your partner's complaints, or do you set the stage for getting what you want? Is it sex on your terms or your partner's terms?

How would you describe your sexual interaction style? Do you see yourself as the cherished one or do you agree to have sex to stop your partner's complaints? Do you fulfill your partner's wishes graciously in return for his admiration of you? Do you regard sex as a service you have to perform or a very special favor that you grant?

Sexual Interaction Style Scale (SISS)

giving	1	2	3	4	3	2	1	taking
passive	1	2	3	4	3	2	1	active, lively
playful	1	2	3	4	3	2	1	serious, quiet
submissive	1	2	3	4	3	2	1	domineering
demanding	1	2	3	4	3	2	1	acquiescent
sacrificing	1	2	3	4	3	2	1	taking advantage
seductive	1	2	3	4	3	2	1	reluctant
joyful	1	2	3	4	3	2	1	resisting
giving in	1	2	3	4	3	2	1	complaining

Please circle the descriptors that apply and mark the level as 1 = very mild to 4 = very strong. Descriptors on the same line appear to be opposites; however, they are not necessarily mutually exclusive. For instance, one can be "giving" and "taking" at different times—or even at the same time. Feel free to add your own descriptors. After going through the rating scales, do you see yourself as "sexually acquiescent" or as assuming the responsibility for getting what you want?

References

Agnew, C. R. (1999). Power over interdependent behavior within the dyad: Who decides what a couple does? In L. J. Sevey & W. Miller (Eds.), *Advances in population: Psychosocial perspectives, Vol. 3* (pp. 162–188). London: Jessica Kingsley Publishers.

Anderson-Hunt, M., & Dennerstein, L. (1995). Oxytocin and female sexuality. *Gynecol Obstet Invest, 40,* 217–221.

Annon, J. S. (1974). *The behavioral treatment of sexual problems: Brief therapy.* New York: Harper & Row.

Antares Pharma. Delivering Promise. (October 23, 2003). Antares Pharma announces its licensee, BioSante Pharmaceuticals, recently presented positive results from Phase II trial of LibiGel™, a topical testosterone gel that utilizes antares pharma's gel technology. Retrieved from the internet http://www.antarespharma.com/content/news/news_10232003, html.

Arentewicz, G., & Schmidt, G. (1983). *The treatment of sexual disorders.* New York: Basic Books, Inc.

Bachmann, G. A. (2004). Strategies for recognition and management of sexual dysfunction in menopausal women. *A Supplement to Contemporary OB/GYN,* September 2004, 4–11.

Balswick, J. O., & Balswick, J. K. (1995). Gender relations and marital power. In B. B. Ingoldsby & S. Smith (Eds.), *Families in multicultural perspective* (pp. 297–313). New York: Guilford.

Bancroft, J. (2002). Biological factors in human sexuality. *The Journal of Sex Research, 39,* 15–21.

Bancroft, J., Loftus, J., & Long, J. (2003). Distress about sex: A national survey of women in heterosexual relationships. *Archives of Sexual Behavior, 32,* 193–209.

Bancroft, J., Sherwin, B. B., Alexander, G. M., Davidson, D. W., & Walker, A. (1991a). Oral contraceptives, androgens, and the sexuality of young women: I. A comparison of sexual experience, sexual attitudes, and gender role in oral contraceptive users and nonusers. *Archives of Sexual Behavior, 20,* 105–119.

Bancroft, J., Sherwin, B. B., Alexander, G. M., Davidson, D. W., & Walker, A. (1991b). Oral contraceptives, androgens, and the sexuality of young women: II. The role of androgens. *Archives of Sexual Behavior, 20,* 121–135.

Barbach, L. (Ed.) (1999). *Seductions: Tales of erotic persuasion.* New York: A Dutton Book.

Barbach, L. (1975/2000). *For Yourself: The fulfillment of female sexuality* (newly revised and updated). New York: Penguin Putnam Books.

Barnard-Jones, K. (1973). A study of two forms of contraception in general practice. *Journal of the Royal College of General Practitioners, 23*, 658–662.

Barrett, G., Pendry, E., Peacock, J., Victor, C., Thakar, R., & Manyonda, I. (1999). Women's sexuality after childbirth: A pilot study. *Archives of Sexual Behavior, 28*, 179–191.

Barrett, G., Pendry, E., Peacock, J., Victor, C., Thakar, R., & Manyonda, I. (2000). Women's sexual health after childbirth. *BJOG: An International Journal of Obstetrics and Gynaecology, 107*, 186–195.

Bart, P. (1993). Protean women: The liquidity of female sexuality and the tenaciousness of lesbian identity. In S. Wilkinson & C. Kitzinger (Eds.), *Heterosexuality: A feminism and psychology reader* (pp. 246–252). London: Sage.

Basson, R. (2000). The female sexual response: A different model. *Journal of Sex & Marital Therapy, 26*, 51–65.

Basson, R. (2001). Female sexual response: The role of drugs in the management of sexual dysfunction. *Obstetrics & Gynecology, 98*, 350–353.

Basson, R. A. (2002). A model of women's sexual arousal. *Journal of Sex and Marital Therapy, 28*, 1–10.

Basson, R. (2003). Commentary on "In the mood for sex"—the value of androgens. *Journal of Sex & Marital Therapy, 29*, 177–179.

Basson, R., Berman, J., Burnett, A., Derogatis, L., Ferguson, D., Fourcroy, J., Goldstein, I., Graziotti, A., Heiman, J., Lann, E., Leiblum, S., Padma-Nathan, H., Rosen, R., Segraves, K., Segraves, T., Shabsigh, R., Sipski, M., Wagner, G., & Whipple, B. (2000). Report of the International Consensus Development Conference on Female Sexual Dysfunction: Definitions and classifications. *Journal of Urology, 163*, 888–893.

Basson, R., McInnes, R., Smith, M. D., Hodgson, G., & Koppiker, N. (2002). Efficacy and safety of sildenafil citrate in women with sexual dysfunction associated with female sexual arousal disorder. *Journal of Womens' Health Gender Based Medicine, 11*, 367–377.

Bateson, M. C. (1989). *Composing a life.* New York: Penguin.

Baumeister, R. F. (2000). Gender differences in erotic plasticity: The female sex drive as socially flexible and responsive. *Psychological Bulletin, 126*, 347–374.

Baumeister, R. F., Catanese, K. R., & Vohs, K. D. (2001). Are there gender differences in strength of sex drive? Theoretical views, conceptual distinctions, and a review of relevant evidence. *Personality and Social Psychology Review, 5*, 242–273.

Baumeister, R. F., & Tice, D. M. (2000). *The social dimension of sex.* New York: Allyn & Bacon.

Baumeister, R. F., & Twenge, J. M. (2002). Cultural suppression of female sexuality. *Review of General Psychology, 6*, 166–203.

Beck, A. T. (1976). *Cognitive therapy and the emotional disorders.* New York: Meridian Books.

Beck, A. T. (1988). *Love is never enough.* New York: Harper & Row Publishers.

Beck, A. T. (1996). Beyond belief: A theory of modes, personality, and psychopathology. In P. Salkovskis (Ed.), *Frontiers of cognitive therapy* (pp. 1–25). New York: Guilford Press.

Becker, G. S. (1991). *A treatise on the family,* 2nd ed. Cambridge, MA: Harvard University Press.

Becker, J., & Kaplan, M. (1991). Rape victims: Issues, theories, and treatment. *Annual Review of Sex Research, 2*, 267–272.

Bentler, P. M., & Speckart, G. (1979). Models of attitude-behavior relations. *Psychological Review, 86*, 452–464.

Berman, L. A., & Berman, J. R. (2000). Viagra and beyond: Where sex educators and therapists fit in from a multidisciplinary perspective. *Journal of Sex Education and Therapy, 25*, 17–24.

Berman, J., Berman, L., & Bumiller, E. (2001). *For women only: A revolutionary guide to overcoming sexual dysfunction and reclaiming your sex life*. New York: Henry Holt and Company.

Berman, L., Berman, J., & Schweiger, A. B. (2005). *Secrets of the sexually satisfied woman: Ten keys to unlocking ultimate pleasure*. New York: Hyperion.

Blumberg, E. S. (2000). The voices of highly sexual women: An orientation to the erotic (Doctoral dissertation, Saybrook Graduate School and Research Center. 2000). *Dissertation Abstracts International, 62*, 5953.

Blumberg, E. S. (2003). The lives and voices of highly sexual women. *The Journal of Sex Research, 40*, 146–157.

Blumstein, P., & Schwartz, P. (1983). *American couples*. New York: William Morrow and Company.

Bogren, L. (1991). Changes in sexuality in women and men during pregnancy. *Archives of Sexual Behavior, 20*, 35–46.

Bowlby, J. (1973). *Attachment and loss: Vol. 2. Separation*. New York: Basic Books.

Bowlby, J. (1980). *Attachment and loss: Vol. 3. Sadness and depression*. New York: Basic Books.

Bowlby, J. (1988). *A secure base*. New York: Basic Books.

Braun, V., & Wilkinson, S. (2001). Socio-cultural representations of the vagina. *Journal of Reproductive and Infant Psychology, 19*, 17–32.

Braunstein, G., Shifren, J., Simon, J., Lucas, J., Rodenberg, C., & Watts, N. (2003). Testosterone patches for the treatment of low sexual desire in surgically menopausal women. *MENOPAUSE, 10*, 70.

Brehm, S. S., Miller, R. S., Perlman, D., & Campbell, S. M. (2002). *Intimate relationships*, 3rd ed. New York: McGraw-Hill.

Brown, J. D. (2002). Mass media influences on sexuality. *The Journal of Sex Research, 39*, 42–45.

Brownmiller, S. (1975). *Against our will: Men, women, and rape*. New York: Simon & Schuster.

Bullough, V. L. (1994). The development of sexology in the USA in the early twentieth century. In R. Porter & M. Teich (Eds.), *Sexual knowledge, sexual science: The history of attitudes to sexuality* (pp. 303–322). New York: Cambridge University Press.

Burleson, M. H., Gregory, W. L., & Trevathan, W. (1991). Heterosexual activity and cycle length variability: Effect of gynecological maturity. *Physiology and Behavior, 50*, 863–866.

BUSINESS WIRE: The Global Leader in News Distribution. BioSante Pharmaceuticals comments on updated FDA guidance for testosterone therapy. November 2, 2005. Retrieved from Internet http://home.businesswire.com/portal/site/home/index.jsp?epi-content=NEWS VIEW POP

Buss, D. (1999). *Evolutionary psychology*. Boston: Allyn & Bacon.

Buster, J. E., Kingsberg, S. A., Aguirre, O., Brown, C., Breaux, J. G., Buch, A., Rodenberg, C. A., Wekselman, K., & Casson, P. (2005). Testosterone patch for low sexual desire in surgically menopausal women: A randomized trial. *OBSTETRICS & GYNECOLOGY, 105*, No. 5 Part 1 (May 2005), 944–952.

Byers, E. S. (2005). Relationship satisfaction and sexual satisfaction: A longitudinal study of individuals in long-term relationships. *The Journal of Sex Research, 42*, 113–118.

Campbell, W. K., & Sedikides, C. (1999). Self-threat magnifies the self-serving bias: A meta-analytic integration. *Review of General Psychology, 3*, 23–43.

Carlson, J. (1976). The sexual role. In F. I. Nye (Ed.), *Role structure and analysis of the family* (pp. 101–110). Beverly Hills, CA: Sage.

Carnes, P. (1983). *Out of the shadows: Understanding sexual addiction.* Minneapolis: Compcare Publications.

Carnes, P. J. (1996). Addiction or compulsion: Politics or illness. *Sexual Addiction & Compulsivity: The Journal of Treatment and Prevention, 3*(2), 127–150.

Carpenter, L. M. (1998). From girls into women: Scripts for sexuality and romance in *Seventeen* magazine, 1974–1994. *The Journal of Sex Research, 35*, 158–168.

Carter, C. S. (1992). Oxytocin and sexual behavior. *Neuroscience and Biobehavioral Reviews, 16*, 131–144.

Cashdan, S. (1988). *Object relations therapy.* New York: W. W. Norton & Company.

Cassell, C. (1984). *Swept away: Why women fear their own sexuality.* New York: Simon and Schuster.

Cervenka, K. A. (2003). *In the mood again.* Oakland, CA: New Harbinger Publications. Inc.

Ciabattari, T. (2001). Changes in men's conservative gender ideologies: Cohort and period influences. *Gender and Society, 15*, 574–591.

Coleman, E. (1995). Treatment of compulsive behavior. In R. C. Rosen & S. R. Leiblum (Eds.), *Case studies in sex therapy* (pp. 333–349). New York: The Guilford Press.

Coleman, E. (2003). Compulsive sexual behavior: What to call it, how to treat it? *SIECUS Report, 31*, 12–16.

Comfort, A. (1972). *The joy of sex.* New York: Crown.

Contemporary Sexuality (1999). Hormone supplements help women regain libido. "Studies in Short," p. 12.

Courtois, C. (2000). The sexual after-effect of incest/child sexual abuse. *SIECUS Report, 29*, 11–16.

Crawford, M., & Popp, D. (2003). Sexual double standards: A review and methodological critique of two decades of research. *Journal of Sex Research, 40*, 13–26.

Crenshaw, T., Goldberg, J., & Stern, W. (1987). Pharmacologic modification of psycho-sexual dysfunction. *Journal of Sex and Marital Therapy, 13*, 239–252.

Crittenden, A. (2001). *The price of motherhood.* New York: Henry Holt and Company.

Cullberg, J. (1972). Mood changes and menstrual symptoms with different gestagen/estrogen combinations. *Acta Psychiatrica Scandinavica, 236* (Suppl.), 1–65.

Cullberg, J., Gelli, M. G., & Jonsson, C. O. (1969). Mental and sexual adjustment before and after six months' use of an oral contraceptive. *Acta Psychiatrica Scandinavica, 45*, 259–276.

Cupach, W. R., & Comstock, J. (1990). Satisfaction with sexual communication in marriage: Links to sexual satisfaction and dyadic adjustment. *Journal of Social and Personal Relationships, 7*, 179–186.

Cutler W. B. (1987). Female essence (pheromones) increases sexual behavior of young women [Abstract]. *Neuroendocrinology Letters, 9*, 199.

Cutler, W. B., Davidson, J. M., & McCoy, N. (1983). Sexual behavior, steroids and hot flashes are associated during the perimenopause. *Neuroendocrinology Letters, 5*, 185.

Cutler, W. B., Friedmann, E., & McCoy, N. L. (1998). Pheromonal influences on socio-sexual behavior in men. *Archives of Sexual Behavior, 27*, 1–13.

Cutler, W. B., Garcia, C. R., Huggins, G. R., & Preti, G. (1986). Sexual behavior and steroid levels among gynecologically mature premenopausal women. *Fertility and Sterility, 45*, 496–502.

Cutler, W. B., & Genovese-Stone, E. G. (2000). Wellness in women after 40: The role of sex hormones and pheromones. (Part I) *Current Problems in Obstetrics, Gynecology and Fertility, 23*, 1–30.

Davidson, J., & Darling, C. (1988). The sexually experienced woman: Multiple sex partners and sexual satisfaction. *The Journal of Sex Research, 24*, 141–154.

Davis, A. R., & Castaño, P. M. (2004). Oral contraceptives and libido in Women. *Annual Review of Sex Research, XV*, 297–320.

Davis, S. R., McCloud, P., Strauss, B. J., & Burger, H. (1995). Testosterone enhances estradiol's effects on postmenopausal bone density and sexuality. *Maturitas, 21*, 227–236.

Degler, C. (1980). *At odds: Women and the family in America from the revolution to the present.* Oxford: Oxford University Press.

De Judicibus, M. A., & McCabe, M. P. (2002). Psychological factors and the sexuality of pregnant and postpartum women. *The Journal of Sex Research, 39*, 94–103.

DeLamater, J. D. (1987). Gender differences in sexual scenarios. In K. Kelley (Ed.), *Females, males and sexuality: Theories and research* (pp. 127–129). Albany, NY: State University of New York Press.

DeLamater, J. D. (1989). The social control of human sexuality. In K. McKinney & S. Sprecher (Eds.), *Human sexuality: The societal and interpersonal context* (pp. 30–62). Norwood, NJ: Ablex.

DeLamater, J., & MacCorquodale, P. (1979). *Premarital sexuality: Attitudes, relationships, behavior.* Madison, WI: University of Wisconsin Press.

DeLamater, J. D., & Sill, M. (2005). Sexual desire in later life. *The Journal of Sex Research, 42*, 138–149.

DeMartino, M. (1970). How women want men to make love. *Sexology*, October, 4–7.

Dennerstein, L., Alexander, J. L., & Kotz, K. (2003). The menopause and sexual functioning: A review of the population-based studies. *Annual Review of Sex Research, 14*, 64–82.

Dennerstein, L., Smith, A. M., Morse, C. A., & Burger, H. G. (1994). Sexuality and the menopause. *Journal of Psychosomatic Obstetrics and Gynaecology, 15*, 59–66.

Derogatis, L. R. (1981). Psychopathology in individuals with sexual dysfunction. *American Journal of Psychiatry, 138*, 757–763.

Diamond, L. M. (2003). Was it a phase? Young women's identities over a 5-year period. *Journal of Personality and Social Psychology, 84*, 352–364.

Diehl, L., Vicary, J., & Deike, R. (1997). Longitudinal trajectories of self-esteem from early to middle adolescence and related psychological variables among rural adolescents. *Journal of Research on Adolescence, 7*, 393–411.

Dodson, B. (1974). *Liberating masturbation.* New York: Betty Dodson.

Dove, N. L., & Wiederman, M. W. (2000). Cognitive distraction and women's sexual functioning. *Journal of Sex & Marital Therapy, 26*, 67–78.

Efthim, P. W., Kenny, M. E., & Mahalik, J. R. (2001). Gender role stress in relation to shame, guilt, and externalization. *Journal of Counseling & Development, 79*, 430–438.

Elliott, A. N., & O'Donohue, W. T. (1997). The effects of anxiety and distraction on sexual arousal in a nonclinical sample of heterosexual women. *Archives of Sexual Behavior, 26*, 607–624.

Ellis, H. (1920). *On life and sex.* Garden City, NY: Garden City Publishing.

Ellison, C. (2000). *Women's sexualities.* Oakland, CA: New Harbinger Publications.

Enserink, M. (2005). Let's talk about sex and drugs. *Science. 308*, 1578 (10 June, in News).

Erikson, E. H. (1950). *Childhood and society.* New York: Norton.

Everaerd, W. (1988). Commentary on sex research: Sex as an emotion. *Journal of Psychology and Human Sexuality, 1*, 3–15.

Farrell, S. A., & Kieser, K. (2000). Sexuality after hysterectomy. *Obstetrics and Gynecology, 95*, 1045–1051.

Farrington, A. (2005). Female sexual health in midlife and beyond: Addressing female sexual distress. *Health & Sexuality, 10*, 2–13.

Feiring, C. (1999). Other-sex friendship networks and the development of romantic relationships in adolescence. *Journal of Youth & Adolescence, 28*, 495–512.

Finkelhor, D., & Browne, A. (1985). The traumatic impact of child sexual abuse: A conceptualization. *American Journal of Orthopsychiatry, 55*, 530–541.

Folb, K. (2000). "Don't touch that dial!" TV as a—what!—positive influence. *SIECUS Report, 28*, 16–18.

Foley, S., Kope, S. A., & Sugrue, D. P. (2002). *Sex matters for women*. New York: The Guilford Press.

Freud, S. (1963). *The standard edition of the complete works of Sigmund Freud* (Vol. 7). London: Hogarth Press.

Fusco, G. M., & Apsche, J. (2005). Cognitive Behavioral therapy. In A. Freeman, M. H. Stone, & D. Martin (Eds.), *Comparative treatments for Borderline Personality Disorder* (pp. 75–103). New York: Springer Publishing Company.

Geary, D. C., Vigil, J., & Byrd-Craven, J. (2004). Evolution of human mate choice. *The Journal of Sex Research, 41*, 27–42.

Gehring, D., & Chan, A. W. C. (2001). Group therapy—a useful treatment modality for women diagnosed with primary and secondary vaginismus. *Journal of Sex Education and Therapy, 26*, 59–67.

Gilbert, L. A., & Walker, S. J. (1999). Dominant discourse in heterosexual relationships: Inhibitors or facilitators of interpersonal commitment and relationship stability? In J. M. Adams & W. H. Jones (Eds.), *Handbook of interpersonal commitment and relationship stability* (pp. 393–406). New York: Kluwer Academic/Plenum.

Ginsburg, E. S., Rosen, R. C., Leiblum, S. R., Caramelli, K. E., & Mazer, N. A. (2000). Transdermal testosterone treatment in women with impaired sexual function after oophorectomy. *The New England Journal of Medicine, 343*, 682–731.

Glick, P., & Fiske, S. (2001). An ambivalent alliance: Hostile and benevolent sexism as complementary justifications for gender inequality. *American Psychologist,* February, 109–118.

Goldzieher, J. W., Moses, L. E., & Ellis, L. T. (1962). Study of norenthindrone in contraception. *Journal of the American Medical Association, 180*, 359–361.

Goleman, D. (1995). *Emotional intelligence*. New York: Bantam.

Graham, B. (1998). *Polyamorous Pollyanna*. Retrieved September 17, 1998, from http/www.phoenixnewtimes.com.

Graham, C. A., Ramos, R., Bancroft, J., Maglaya, C., & Farley, T. M. (1995). The effects of steroidal contraceptives on the well-being and sexuality of women: A double-blind, placebo-controlled, two-centre study of combined and progestogen-only methods. *Contraception, 52*, 363–369.

Graham, C. A., Sanders, S. A., Milhausen, R. R., & McBride, K. R. (2004). Turning on and turning off: A focus group study of the factors that affect women's sexual arousal. *Archives of Sexual Behavior, 33*, 527–538.

Graham, C. A., & Sherwin, B. B. (1993). The relationship between mood and sexuality in women using an oral contraceptive as a treatment for premenstrual symptoms. *Psychoneuroendocrinology, 18*, 273–281.

Greenberg, B., & Busselle, R. (1996). Soap operas and sexual activity: A decade later. *Journal of Communication, 46*, 153–161.

Guay, A. T. (2002). Screening for androgen deficiency in women: Methodological and interpretive issues. *Fertility and Sterility, 77* (Suppl. 4) S83–88.

Hajcak, F., & Garwood, P. (1987). *Hidden bedroom partners: Needs and motives that destroy sexual pleasure.* San Diego, CA: Libra Publishers, Inc.

Halgin, R. P., Hennessey, J. E., Statlender, S., Feinman, J. A., & Bown, R. A. (1988). Treatment of sexual dysfunction in the context of general psychotherapy. In R. A. Brown & J. R. Field (Eds.), *Treatment of sexual problems in individual and couples therapy* (pp. 3–21). PMA Publishing Corp.

Hall, L. A. (1994). The English have hot-water bottles: the morganatic marriage between sexology and medicine in Britain since William Acton. In R. Porter & M. Teich (Eds.), *Sexual knowledge, sexual science: The history of attitudes to sexuality* (pp. 350–366). Cambridge: Cambridge University Press.

Harris, A. (1985). *Sexual exercises for women.* New York: Carroll & Graf Publishers, Inc.

Hartman, W. E., & Fithian, M. A. (1974) *Treatment of sexual dysfunction.* New York: Jason Aronson.

Harvey, S. M., Beckman, L. J., Browner, C. H., & Sherman, C. A. (2002). Relationship power, decision making, and sexual relations: An exploratory study with couples of Mexican origin. *The Journal of Sex Research, 39*, 284–291.

Hauch, M. (1998). The Hamburg Model: Couples therapy at century's end. *Journal of Sex Education and Therapy, 23*, 237–245.

Hauser, R. (1994). Krafft-Ebing's psychological understanding of sexual behaviour. In R. Porter & M. Teich (Eds.), *Sexual knowledge, sexual science: The history of attitudes to sexuality* (pp. 210–227). Cambridge: Cambridge University Press.

Heiman, Julia R. (2002). Sexual dysfunction: Overview of prevalence, etiological factors, and treatments. *The Journal of Sex Research, 39*, 73–78.

Herzberg, B. N., Draper, K. C., Johnson, A. L., & Nicol, G. C. (1971). Oral contraceptives, depression, and libido. *British Medical Journal, 3*, 495–500.

Heyn, D. (1997). *Marriage shock: The transformation of women into wives.* New York: Villard Books.

Hite, S. (1976). *The Hite report: A nationwide study of female sexuality.* New York: Dell.

Hyde, J. S., & DeLamater, J. (1997). *Understanding human sexuality* (6th ed.). Boston: McGraw-Hill.

Impett, E. A., & Peplau, L. A. (2000, August). *Saying "yes" but thinking "no": Consensual participation in unwanted sex.* Paper presented at the annual meeting of the American Psychological Association, Washington, DC.

Impett, E. A., & Peplau, L. A. (2002). Why some women consent to unwanted sex with a dating partner: Insights from attachment theory. *Psychology of Women Quarterly, 26*, 359–369.

Impett, E. A., & Peplau, L. A. (2003). Sexual compliance: Gender, motivational, and relationship perspectives. *The Journal of Sex Research, 40*, 87–100.

Insel, T. R. (1997). A neurobiological basis of social attachment. *The American Journal of Psychiatry, 154*(6), 726–735.

Jacoby, S. (2005). Sex in America. *AARP The Magazine, 48*, 55–58, 82.

James, W. H. (1983). Decline in coital rates with spouses' ages and duration of marriage. *Journal of Biosocial Science, 15*, 83–87.

Kaplan, H. S. (1974). *The new sex therapy: Active treatment of sexual dysfunctions.* New York: Brunner/Mazel.

Kaplan, H. S. (1977). Hypoactive sexual desire. *Journal of Sex and Marital Therapy, 3*, 3–9.

Kaplan, H. S. (1979). *Disorders of sexual desire*. New York: Brunner/Mazel.

Kaplan, H. S. (1995). *The sexual desire disorders*. New York: Brunner/Mazel.

Keller Ashton, A., Hamer, R., & Rosen, R. C. (1997). Serotonin reuptake inhibitor-induced sexual dysfunction and its treatment: A large-scale retrospective study of 596 psychiatric outpatients. *Journal of Sex & Marital Therapy, 23*, 165–175.

Kelman, H. C. (1974). Attitudes are alive and well and gainfully employed in the sphere of action. *American Psychologist, 29*, 310–324.

Kimmel, M. S. (2000). *The gendered society*. New York: Oxford University Press.

Kingsberg, S.A. (2005). Hypoactive sexual desire disorder in postmenopausal women: Psychologic aspects. *OBG Management*, Supplement, March 2005, 2–9.

Kinsey, A., Pomeroy, W., & Martin, C. (1948). *Sexual behavior in the human male*. Philadelphia: Saunders.

Kinsey, A., Pomeroy, W., Martin, C., & Gebhard, P. (1953). *Sexual behavior in the human female*. Philadelphia: Saunders.

Kitzinger, C., & Wilkinson, S. (1995). Transition from heterosexuality to lesbianism: The discursive production of lesbian identities. *Developmental Psychology, 31*, 95–104.

Klein, M. (2003). Sex addiction: A dangerous clinical concept. *SIECUS Report, 31*, 8–11.

Kleinke, C. L. (1978). *Self-perception: The psychology of personal awareness*. San Francisco: Freedman.

Klusmann, D. (2002). Sexual motivation and the duration of partnership. *Archives of Sexual Behavior, 31*, 275–287.

Koch, P. B. (1998). Current developments. In R. T. Francoeur, P. B. Koch, & D. L. Weis (Eds.), *Sexuality in America: Understanding our sexual values and behavior* (pp. 278–281). New York: Continuum.

Koch, P. B., Mansfield, P. K., Thurau, D., & Carey, M. (2005). "Feeling frumpy": The relationships between body image and sexual response changes in midlife women. *The Journal of Sex Research, 42*, 215–223.

Koehler, J., Zangwill, W., & Lotz, L. (2000). *Integrating the power of EMDR into sex therapy*. Paper presented at the 32nd Annual Conference of the American Association of Sex Educators, Counselors, and Therapists, Atlanta, GA, May 10–14.

Krafft-Ebing, R., von (1902) *Psychosis menstrualis. Eine klinisch-forensische Studie* (A clinico-forensic study). Stuttgart: Enke.

Kurcinka, M. S. (2000). *Kids, parents, and power struggles*. New York: HarperCollins.

Kuriansky, J. B. (1988). Personality style and sexuality. In R. A. Brown, & J. R. Field (Eds.), *Treatment of sexual problems in individual and couples therapy*. (pp. 23–47). PMA Publishing Corp.

Kuypers, J. A. (1999a) The paradox of men's power. In J. A. Kuypers (Ed.), *Men and power* (pp. 17–33). Amherst, NY: Prometheus Books.

Kuypers, J. A. (Ed.) (1999b). Introduction. In J. A. Kuypers (Ed.), *Men and power* (pp. 7–11). Amherst, NY: Prometheus Books.

Laumann, E. O., Gagnon, J. H., Michael, R. T., & Michaels, S. (1994). *The social organization of sexuality*. Chicago: University of Chicago Press.

Laumann, E. O., Paik, A., & Rosen, R. C. (1999). Sexual dysfunction in the United States: Prevalence and predictors. *JAMA: The Journal of the American Medical Association, 281*, 537–544.

Lawrance, K., & Byers, E. S. (1995). Sexual satisfaction in long-term heterosexual relationships: The Interpersonal Exchange Model of Sexual Satisfaction. *Personal Relationships, 2*, 267–285.

Leckman, J. F., Goodman, W. K., North, W. G., Chappell, P. B., Price, L. H., Pauls, D. L., Anderson, G. M., Riddle, M. A., McDougle, C. J., Barr, L. C., & Cohen, D. J. (1994). The role of central oxytocin in obsessive compulsive disorder and related normal behavior. *Psychoneuroendocrinology, 19*(8), 723–749.

Leedes, Richard (1999). Theory and praxis: A heuristic for describing, evaluating, and intervening on sexual desire disorders when sexual expression interferes with humanistic expression. *Sexual Addiction & Compulsivity:The Journal of Treatment and Prevention, 6*(4), 289–310.

Leeton, J., McMaster, R., & Worsley, A. (1978). The effects on sexual response and mood after sterilization of women taking long-term oral contraception: Results of a double-blind cross-over study. *Australia and New Zealand Journal of Obstetrics and Gynecology, 18*, 194–197.

Leiblum, S. R., & Rosen, R. C. (1988). Introduction: Changing perspectives on sexual desire. In S. R. Leiblum & R. C. Rosen (Eds.), *Sexual desire* (pp. 1–17). New York: The Guilford Press.

Leiblum, S. R., & Rosen, R. C. (1989). Introduction: Sex therapy in the age of AIDS. In S. R. Leiblum & R. C. Rosen (Eds.), *Principles and practice of sex therapy* (pp. 1–16). New York: The Guilford Press.

Leiblum, S., & Sachs, J. (2002). *Getting the sex you want: A woman's guide to becoming proud, passionate, and pleased in bed.* New York: Crown Publishers.

Leidy-Sievert, L., Waddle, D., & Canali, K. (2001). Marital status and age at natural menopause: Considering pheromonal influence. *American Journal of Human Biology, 13*, 479–485.

Leitenberg, H., & Henning, K. (1995). Sexual fantasy. *Psychological Bulletin, 117*, 469–496.

Levin, S. (1987). More on the nature of sexual desire. *Journal of Sex & Marital Therapy,13*, 35–44.

Levine, S. (1992). *Sexual life.* New York: Plenum Press.

Levine, S. B. (1997). Some reflections on countertransference: A discussion of Dr. Derek Polonsky's presentation. *Journal of Sex Education and Therapy, 22*, 13–17.

Libido Drug Update: Cold Shower from FDA, January 2005, *AARP Bulletin,46*, 21. INSIDEDOPE Section.

Lief, H. (1977). Inhibited sexual desire. *Medical Aspects of Human Sexuality, 7*, 94–95.

Lips, H. M. (2005). *Sex and gender: An introduction* (5th edition). New York: McGraw-Hill.

Lobo, R. A., Bachmann, G. A., Carey, J. C., Gass, M. L. S., Hutcherson, H., Kingsberg, S. A., & Simon, J. A. (2005). Considerations in evaluating, diagnosing, and treating HSDD in postmenopausal women. *CONTEMPORARY OB/GYN,* Supplement, April 2005, 4–12.

Lobo, R. A., Rosen, R. C., Yang, H. M., Block, B., & Van Der Hoop, R. G. (2003). Comparative effects of oral esterified estrogens with and without methyltestosterone on endocrine profiles and dimensions of sexual function in postmenopausal women with hypoactive sexual desire. *Fertility and Sterility, 79*, 1341–1352.

LoPiccolo, J. (2000, May). *Post-modern sex therapy: An integrated approach.* Paper presented at the 32nd Annual Conference of the American Association of Sex Educators, Counselors, and Therapists, Atlanta, Georgia.

LoPiccolo, J., & Friedman, J. (1988). Broad-spectrum treatment of low sexual desire: Integration of cognitive, behavioral, and systemic therapy. In S. Leiblum & R. Rosen (Eds.), *Sexual desire disorders* (pp. 107–144). New York: Guilford Press.

Lytle, L., Bakken, L., & Romig, C. (1997). Adolescent female identity development. *Sex Roles, 37*, 175–185.

Maas, C. P., Kenter, G. G., & Trimbos, J. B. (2003). Outcomes after total versus subtotal abdominal hysterectomy [Letter to the Editor]. *New England Journal of Medicine, 348*, 856–857.

Maas, C. P., Weijenborg, P. T., & ter Kuile, M. M. (2003). The effect of hysterectomy on sexual functioning. *Annual Review of Sex Research, 14*, 83–113.

Maass, V. S. (2000, May). *The function and impact of attention throughout life.* Paper presented at the 2000 Spring Convention of the Indiana Psychological Association, South Bend, IN.

Maass, V. S. (2002) *Women's group therapy: Creative challenges and options.* New York: Springer Publishing Company.

Maass, V. S. (2005). Single-sided relationship therapy: An alternative. AFTA-IFTA 2005, The International Conference on Family Therapy, Washington, DC, June 22–25, 2005.

Maass, V. S. (2006). Images of masculinity as predictors of men's romantic and sexual relationships. In V. H. Bedford & B. F. Turner (Eds.), *Men in relationships: A new look from a life course perspective* (pp. 51–78). New York: Springer Publishing Company.

Maass, V. S., & Neely, M. A. (2000). *Counseling single parents: A cognitive-behavioral approach.* New York: Springer Publishing Company.

MacNeil, S., & Byers, E. S. (2005). Dyadic assessment of sexual self-disclosure and sexual satisfaction. *Journal of Personal and Social Relationships, 22*, 193–205.

Mahoney, S. (2003). Seeking love: The 50-plus dating game has never been hotter. *AARP*, November-December, 57–66.

Marcia, J. E. (1966). Development and validation of ego identity status. *Journal of Personality and Social Psychology, 3*, 551–558.

Marcia, J. E. (1980). Identity in adolescence. In J. Adelson (Ed.), *Handbook of adolescent psychology* (pp. 159–187). New York: Wiley.

Massafra, C., De Felice, C., Agnusdei, D. P., Gioia, D., & Bagnoli, F. (1999). Androgens and osteocalcin during the menstrual cycle. *Journal of Clini. Endocrinol. Metab., 84*, 971–974.

Masters, W., & Johnson, V. (1966). *Human sexual response.* Boston: Little, Brown.

Masters, W., & Johnson, V. (1970). *Human sexual inadequacy.* Boston: Little, Brown.

Masters, W., Johnson, V., & Kolodny, R. (1994). *Heterosexuality.* New York: Harper Collins.

May, L. (1998). *Masculinity & morality.* Ithaca, NY: Cornell University Press.

McCarthy, B., & MacCarthy, E. (2003). *Rekindling desire: A step-by-step program to help low-sex and no-sex marriages.* New York: Brunner-Routledge.

McCarthy, B. W., Ryan, M., & Johnson, F. A. (1975). *Sexual awareness: A practical approach.* San Francisco: Boyd & Fraser Publishing Company, The Scrimshaw Press, Inc.

McCoy, N. L. (1998). Methodological problems in the study of the effects of menopause on sexuality. *Maturitas, 7*, 203–210.

McCoy, N., Cutler, W. B., & Davidson, J. M. (1985). Relationships among sexual behavior, hot flashes, and hormone levels in perimenopausal women. *Archives of Sexual Behavior, 14*, 385–394.

McCoy, N., & Pitino, L. (2002). Pheromonal influences on sociosexual behavior in young women. *Physiology and Behavior, 75*, 367–375.

McCracken, E. (1993). *Decoding women's magazines: From Mademoiselle to Ms.* London: MacMillan Press.

McCrone, J. (1993). *The myth of irrationality*. New York: Carroll & Graf.

McDonald, D. (2004). Conrad wanted more. *Vanity Fair,* April, 2004, 290–339.

McKee, A. (2005). The objectification of women in mainstream pornographic videos in Australia. *The Journal of Sex Research, 42,* 277–290.

McKinlay, J., & Feldman, H. (1994). Age-related variations in sexual activity and interest in normal men: Results from the Massachusetts Male Aging Study. In A. S. Rossi (Ed.), *Sexuality across the life course* (pp. 261–285). Chicago: University of Chicago Press.

McKinley, N. M. (2002). Feminist perspectives and objectified body consciousness. In T. F. Cash & T. Pruzinsky (Eds.), *Body image* (pp. 55–64). New York: Guilford Press.

McRobbie A. (1991). *Feminism and youth culture: From Jackie to Just Seventeen.* Cambridge, MA: Unwin Hyman.

Merriwether, A., & Ward, L. M. (2002, August). *Comfort in our skin: The impact of women's reproductive attitudes*. Poster presented at the annual meeting of the American Psychological Association, Chicago.

Meston, C. M., Heiman, J. R., & Trapnell, P. D. (1999). The relation between early abuse and adult sexuality. *The Journal of Sex Research, 36,* 385–395.

Michael, R., Gagnon, J., Laumann, E., & Kolata, G. (1994). *Sex in America*. Boston: Little, Brown.

Michelson, D., Schmidt, M., Lee, J., & Tepner, R. (2001). Changes in sexual function during acute and six-month fluoxetine therapy: A prospective assessment. *Journal of Sex & Marital Therapy, 27,* 289–302.

Millhausen, R. R., & Herold, E. S. (1999). Does the sexual double standard still exist? *Journal of Sex Research, 36,* 361–368.

Minkin, M. J., & Wright, C. V. (1996). *What every woman needs to know about menopause*. New Haven, CT: Yale University Press.

Money, J. (1986). *Lovemaps: Clinical concepts of sexual/erotic health and pathology, paraphilia, and gender transposition in childhood, adolescence, and maturity*. New York: Irvington Publishers.

Montejo, A. L., Llorca, G., Izquierdo, J. A., & Rico-Villademoros, F. (2001). Incidence of sexual dysfunction associated with antidepressant agents: A prospective multicenter study of 1022 outpatients. Spanish Working Group for the Study of Psychotropic-Related Sexual Dysfunction. *The Journal of Clinical Psychiatry, 62* (Suppl. 3), 10–21.

Montgomery, M., & Sorel, G. (1997). Differences in love attitudes across family life stages. *Family Relations, 46,* 55–61.

Moretti, M., & Wiebe, V. (1999). Self-discrepancy in adolescence: Own and parental standpoints on the self. *Merrill-Palmer Quarterly, 45,* 624–649.

Morse, J. M., Kieren, D., & Bottorff, J. (1993). The Adolescent Menstrual Attitude Questionnaire: I. Scale construction. *Health Care for Women International, 14*(1), 39–62.

Muehlenhard, C. L., & McCoy, M. L. (1991). Double standard/double bind: The sexual double standard and women's communication about sex. *Psychology of Women Quarterly, 15,* 447–461.

Muehlenhard, C. L., & Schrag, J. L. (1991). Nonviolent sexual coercion. In A. Parrot & L. Bechhofer (Eds.), *Acquaintance rape: The hidden crime* (pp. 115–128). New York: Wiley.

National Council on Sexual Addiction and Compulsivity (2002). Information statement: Women sex addicts. *Sexual Addiction and Compulsivity, 9,* 293–295.

Nobre, P. J., & Pinto-Gouveia, J. (2003). Sexual modes questionnaire: Measure to assess the interaction among cognitions, emotions and sexual response. *The Journal of Sex Research, 40,* 368–382.

Oboro, V. O., & Tabowei, T. O. (2002). Sexual function after childbirth in Nigerian women. *International Journal of Gynaecology and Obstetrics, 78*, 249–250.

Ogden, G. (1990) Sexual recovery: Everywoman's guide through sexual co-dependency. Deerfield Beach, FA: Health Communications, Inc.

O'Leary, K. D., & Arias, N. (1983). The influence of marital therapy on sexual satisfaction. *Journal of Sex and Marital Therapy, 9*, 171–181.

Oliver, M. B., & Hyde, J. S. (1993). Gender differences in sexuality: A meta-analysis. *Psychological Bulletin, 114*, 29–51.

O'Sullivan, L. F., & Allgeier, E. R. (1998). Feigning sexual desire: Consenting to unwanted sexual activity in heterosexual dating relationships. *The Journal of Sex Research, 35*, 234–243.

Pertot, S. (2005). *Perfectly normal: Living and loving with low libido.* Emmaus, PA:Rodale, Inc.

Pillsworth, E. G., Haselton, M. G., & Buss, D. M. (2004). Ovulatory shifts in female sexual desire. *The Journal of Sex Research, 41*, 55–65.

Pipher, M. (1994). *Reviving Ophelia: Saving the selves of adolescent girls.* New York: Ballantine Books.

Pittman, F. S. III (1993). *Man enough: Fathers, sons, and the search for masculinity.* New York: G. P. Putnam's Sons.

Planned Parenthood Federation of America (2001). *White paper: Adolescent sexuality.* New York: Author.

Polonsky, D. C. (1997). What do you do when they won't do it? The therapist's dilemma with low desire. *Journal of Sex Education and Therapy, 22*, 5–12.

Rabe, T., Kowald, A., Ortman, J., & Rehberger-Schneider, S. (2000). Inhibition of skin 5 alpha-reductase by oral contraceptive progestins in vitro. *Gynecological Endocrinology, 14*, 223–230.

Rako, S., & Friebely, J. (2004). Pheromonal influences on sociosexual behavior in postmenopausal women. *The Journal of Sex Research, 41*, 372–380.

Redmond, G. P., Olson, W. H., Lippman, J. S., Kafrisen, M. E., Jones, T. M., & Jorizzo, J. L. (1997). Norgestimate and ethinyl estradiol in the treatment of acne vulgaris: A randomized, placebo-controlled trial. *Obstetrics and Gynecology, 89*, 615–622.

Regan, P. C., & Berscheid, E. (1999). *Lust: What we know about sexual desire.* Thousand Oaks, CA: Sage Publications.

Reinholtz, R. K., & Muehlenhard, C. L. (1995). Genital perceptions and sexual activity in a college population. *The Journal of Sex Research, 32*, 155–165.

Reinisch, J. M., & Beasley, R. (1990). *The Kinsey Institute new report on sex: What you must know to be sexually literate.* New York: St. Martin's Press.

Reiss, I. L. (1967). *The social context of premarital sexual permissiveness.* New York: Holt, Rinehart & Winston.

Rempel, J., & Baumgartner, B. (2003). The relationship between attitudes towards menstruation and sexual attitudes, desires, and behavior in women. *Archives of Sexual Behavior, 32*, 155–163.

Reiter, R., & Milburn, A. (1994, March). Exploring effective treatment for chronic pelvic pain. *Contemporary OB/GYN*, 84–103.

Rhodes, J. C., Kjerulff, K. H., Langenberg, P. W., & Guzingski, G. M. (1999). Hysterectomy and sexual functioning. *JAMA: The Journal of the American Medical Association, 282*, 1934–1941.

Richard, D. (2000). Christian women have more fun, study finds. *Contemporary Sexuality, 34* (June 2000) pp. 1, 4.

Riggio, R. E. (1987). *The charisma quotient.* New York: Dodd, Mead & Company.

Rosen, R. C., Lane, R. M., & Menza, M. (1999). Effects of SSRIs on sexual function: A critical review. *Journal of Clinical Psychopharmacology, 19,* 67–85.

Rosen, R. C., & Leiblum, S. R. (1995). The changing focus of sex therapy. In R. C. Rosen & S. R. Leiblum (Eds.), *Case studies in sex therapy* (pp. 3–17). New York: The Guilford Press.

Rosen, R. C., Taylor, J. F., Leiblum, S. R., & Bachmann, G. A. (1993). Prevalence of sexual dysfunction in women: Results of a survey study of 329 women in an outpatient gynecological clinic. *Journal of Sex & Marital Therapy, 19,* 171–188.

Rossouw, J. E., Anderson, G. L., Prentice, R. L., LaCroix, A. Z., Kooperberg, C., Stefanick, M. L., Jackson, R. D., Beresford, S. A., Howard, B. V., Johnson, K. C., Kotchen, J. M., & Ockene, J. (2002). Writing Group for the Women's Health Initiative Investigators. Risks and benefits of estrogen plus progestin in healthy postmenopausal women: Principal results from the Women's Health Initiative. *JAMA: The Journal of the American Medical Association, 288,* 321–333.

Rubin, L. (1990). *Erotic wars: What happened to the sexual revolution?* New York: Farrar, Straus & Giroux.

Russell, M. J., Switz, G. M., & Thompson, K. (1980). Olfactory influences on the human menstrual cycle. *Pharmacology, Biochemistry and Behavior, 13,* 737–738.

Rust, P. C. (1992). The politics of sexual identity: Sexual attraction and behavior among lesbian and bisexual women. *Social Problems, 39,* 366–386.

Rutter, P. (1989). *Sex in the forbidden zone: When men in power—therapists, doctors, clergy, teachers, and others—betray women's trust.* New York: Fawcett Crest.

Rychlak, J. F. (1973). *Introduction to personality and psychotherapy: A theory-construction approach.* Boston: Houghton Mifflin Company.

Sabatelli, R. M. & Shehan, C. L. (1993). Exchange in resources theories. In P. Boss et al. (Eds.), *Sourcebook of family theories and methods* (pp. 385–411). New York: Plenum.

Saks, B. R. (2000). Sex receptors: Mechanisms of drug action via biochemical receptors on sexual response of women. *Journal of Sex Education and Therapy, 25,* 33–35.

Samuels, A., Croal, N., & Gates, D. (2000). Battle for the soul of hiphop. *Newsweek,* October 9, 57–66.

Sanders, S., Graham, C., Bass, J., & Bancroft, J. (2001). A prospective study of the effects of oral contraceptives on sexuality and well-being and their relationship to discontinuation. *Contraception, 64,* 51–58.

Sarrel, P., Dobay, B., & Wiita, B. (1998). Estrogen and estrogen-androgen replacement in postmenopausal women dissatisfied with estrogen-only therapy. Sexual behavior and neuroendocrine responses. *Journal of Reproductive Medicine, 43,* 847–856.

Sattel, J. W. (1983) Men, inexpressiveness, and power. In B. Thorne, C. Kramarae, & N. Henley (Eds.). *Language, gender and society* (pp. 118–124). New York: Newbury House Publishers, A Division of Harper & Row, Publishers, Inc.

Sayers, J. (1991). *Mothers of psychoanalysis.* New York: W. W. Norton.

Sayle, A. E., Savitz, D. A., Thorp, J M. J., Hertz-Picciotto, I., & Wilcox, A. J. (2001). Sexual activity during late pregnancy and risk of preterm delivery. *Obstetrics and Gynecology, 97,* 283–289.

Schnarch, D. (1997). *Passionate marriage.* New York: W. W. Norton & Company.

Schneider, J. P. (1994). Sexual addiction: Controversy in mainstream addiction medicine, diagnosis based on the DSM-III-R and physician case histories. *Sexual Addiction & Compulsivity, 1,* 17–45.

Schooler, D. (2001). *Messages about menstruation: The role of menstrual education in shaping young women's attitudes about menstruation and their sexual decision making.* Unpublished Master's Thesis, University of Michigan.

Schooler, D., Ward, L. M., Merriwether, A., & Caruthers, A. S. (2005). Cycles of shame: Menstrual shame, body shame, and sexual decision-making. *The Journal of Sex Research, 42,* 324–334.

Schwartz, M. F., & Masters, W. H. (1994). Integration of trauma-based, cognitive, behavioral, systemic and addiction approaches for treatment of hypersexual pair-bonding disorder. *Sexual Addiction & Compulsivity, 1,* 6–18.

Seidman, S. N., & Rieder, R. O. (1994). A review of sexual behavior in the United States. *American Journal of Psychiatry, 151,* 330–341.

Shainess, N. (1984). *Sweet suffering: Woman as victim.* Indianapolis/New York: Bobbs-Merrill.

Shapiro, F. (1995). Remarks presented at the opening ceremony of the International EMDR Conference, Santa Monica, California, June 23–25.

Sherwin, B. B., & Gelfand, M. M. (1987). The role of androgen in the maintenance of sexual functioning in oophorectomized women. *Psychosomatic Medicine, 49,* 397–409.

Shifren, J., Braunstein, G., Simon, J., Casson, P., Buster, J., Redmond, G., Burki, R., Ginsburg, E., Jones, K., Rosen, R., Leiblum, S., Daugherty, C., Caramelli, K., & Mazer, N. (2000) Transdermal testosterone treatment in women with impaired sexual function after oophorectomy. *New England Journal of Medicine, 343,* 682–688.

Shokrollahi, P., Mirmohamadi, M., Mehrabi, F., & Babaei, G. (1999). Prevalence of sexual dysfunction in women seeking services at family planning centers in Tehran. *Journal of Sex & Marital Therapy, 25,* 211–215.

Shotland, R. L., & Hunter, B. A. (1995). Women's token resistant and compliant sexual behaviors are related to uncertain sexual intentions and rape. *Personality and Social Psychology Bulletin, 21,* 226–236.

Siddle, N., Sarrel, P., & Whitehead, M. (1987). The effects of hysterectomy on the age at ovarian failure: Identification of a subgroup of women with premature loss of ovarian function and literature review. *Fertility & Sterility, 47,* 94–100.

Simon, J. A. (2004). Emerging treatment strategies for menopausal women with HSDD: The role of testosterone therapy. *A Supplement to CONTEMPORARY OB/GYN,* September 2004, 18–23.

Simon, J. A. (2005). Restoring sexual desire after surgical menopause: Update on assessment and management. *Current Women's Health Reviews, 1,* 143–149.

Simon, J., Braunstein, G., Nachtigall, L., Utian, W., Katz, M., Miller, S., Waldbaum, A., Bouchard, C., Derzko, D., Buch, A., Rodenberg, C., Lucas, J., & Davis, S. (2005). Testosterone patch increases sexual activity and desire in surgically menopausal women with hypoactive sexual desire disorder. *The Journal of Clinical Endocrinology & Metabolism, 90*(9), 5226–5233.

Simon, J., Davis, S., Rees, M., Eymer, V., Moufarege, A., Braunstein, G., Purdie, D., & Ribot, C. (2003). Safety of testosterone patches in surgically menopausal women. *Maturitas, 44,* Supplement 2, S105–S106.

Simon, J. A., Davis, S. R., Watts, N. B., Eymer, V. P., Lucas, J. D., & Braunstein, G. D. (2002). Safety and tolerability of transdermal testosterone therapy versus placebo in surgically menopausal women receiving oral or transdermal estrogen. *MENOPAUSE, 9,* 87.

Simon, W. (1994). Deviance as history: The future of perversion. *Archives of Sexual Behavior, 23,* 1–20.

Spark, R. F. (2005). Intrinsa fails to impress FDA advisory panel. *International Journal of Impotence Research, 17,* 283–284.

Sprecher, S., & Toro-Morn, M. (2002). A study of men and women from different sides of earth to determine if men are from mars and women are from venus in their beliefs about love and romantic relationships. *Sex Roles: A Journal of Research* (March):131–148.

Stern, K., & McClintock, M. K. (1998). Regulation of ovulation by human pheromones [Letter to the editor]. *Nature, 392,* 177–179.

Tannen, D. (1994). *Gender and discourse.* New York: Oxford University Press.

Tays, T. M., Earle, R. H., Wells, K., Murray, M., & Garrett, B. (1999). Treating sex offenders using the sex addiction model. *Sexual Addiction & Compulsivity, 6,* 281–288.

The Working Group for a New View of Women's Sexual Problems (Alperstein, L., Ellison, C., Fishman, J. R., Hall, M., Handwerker, L., Hartley, H., Kaschak, E., Kleinplatz, P., Loe, M., Mamo, L., Tavris, C., & Tiefer, L.) (2001). A new view of women's sexual problems. In E. Kaschak & L. Tiefer (Eds.) *A new view of women's sexual problems* (pp. 1–8). New York: The Haworth Press, Inc.

Tiefer, L. (2001). Arriving at a "new view" of women's sexual problems: Background, theory, and activism. In E. Kaschak & L. Tiefer (Eds.), *A new view of women's sexual problems* (pp. 63–98). New York: The Haworth Press, Inc.

Tiefer, L. (2004) *Sex is not a natural act* (2nd Edition). Boulder, CO: Westview Press.

Thakar, R., Ayers, S., Clarkson, P., Stanton, S., & Manyonda, I. (2002). Outcomes after total versus subtotal abdominal hysterectomy. *New England Journal of Medicine, 347,* 1318–1325.

Thompson, S. (1995). *Going all the way: Teenage girls' tales of sex, romance, and pregnancy.* New York: Hill and Wang.

Tolman, D. L. (1994). Doing desire: Adolescent girls' struggles for/with sexuality. *Gender and Society, 8,* 324–342.

Tolman, D. L. (2000). *Gender equity and adolescent outcomes in a middle school environment.* (Final Rep. to the Spencer Foundation Small Grants Program). Wellesley, MA: Wellesley College, Center for Research on Women.

Tolman, D. L. (2001). Female adolescent sexuality: An argument for a developmental perspective on the new view of women's sexual problems. In E. Kaschak & L. Tiefer (Eds.), *A new view of women's sexual problems* (pp. 195–209). New York: The Haworth Press, Inc.

Trapnell, P. D., Meston, C. M., & Gorzalka, B. B. (1997). Spectatoring and the relationship between body image and sexual experience: Self focus or self valence? *Journal of Sex Research, 34,* 267–278.

Travis, C. B., & White, J. W. (Eds.) (2000). *Sexuality, society, and feminism.* Washington, DC: American Psychological Association.

Trudel, G., Marchand, A., Ravart, M., Aubin, S., Turgeon, I., & Fortier, P. (2001). The effect of a cognitive-behavioral group treatment program on hypoactive sexual desire in women. *Sexual and Relationship Therapy, 16,* 145–164.

U. S. Census Bureau. 2000. *Statistical Abstract of the United States,* 120th ed. Washington, DC: Government Printing Office. www.census.gov/stat_abstract.

Vance, C. V. (1989). *Pleasure and danger: Exploring female sexuality.* London: Pandora.

Verhulst, J., & Heiman, J. (1979). An interactional approach to sexual dysfunctions. *American Journal of Family Therapy, 7,* 19–36.

Vliet, E. L. (2005). *The savvy woman's guide to testosterone.* Tucson, AZ: HER Place Press.

Walen, S. R. (1980). Cognitive factors in sexual behavior. *Journal of Sex and Marital Therapy, 6,* 87–101.

Warner, R. E. (1991). Canadian university counselors: A survey of theoretical orientations and other related descriptors. *Canadian Journal of Counselling/Revue Canadienne de Counseling, 25*(1), 33–37.

Wells, B. E., & Twenge, J. M. (2005). Changes in young people's sexual behavior and attitudes, 1943–1999: A cross-temporal meta-analysis. *Review of General Psychology, 9*, 249–261.

West, S. L., Vinikoor, L. C., & Zolnoun, D. (2004). A systematic review of the literature on female sexual dysfunction prevalence and predictors. *Annual Review of Sex Research, XV*, 40–172.

Westerlund, E. (1992). *Women's sexuality after childhood incest.* New York: W. W. Norton.

Whipple, B. (2002). Women's sexual pleasure and satisfaction: A new view of female sexual function. *The Female Patient, 27*, 39–44.

Whipple, B., & Brash McGreer, K. (1997). Management of female sexual dysfunction. In: M. L. Sipski, and C. J. Alexander (Eds.), *Sexual function in people with disability and chronic illness. A health professional's guide* (pp. 509–534). Gaithersburg, MD: Aspen Publishers, Inc.

Whisnant, P. S., Hammond, R., & Tilmon, R. (1999). Comparing methods of counseling among Arkansas CADCs. *The Counselor, 17*, 33–36.

Wiederman, M. (2000). Women's body image self-consciousness during physical intimacy with a partner. *Journal of Sex Research, 37*, 60–68.

Williams, J. H. (1983). *Psychology of women: Behavior in a biosocial context* (Second edition). New York: W. W. Norton & Company.

Wollstonecraft, M. (1792). *The vindication of the rights of women.* Boston: Peter Edes/Thomas & Andrews.

Woody, J., Russel, R., D'Souza, H., & Woody, J. (2000). Noncoital sex among adolescent virgins and nonvirgins. *Journal of Sex Education and Therapy, 25*, 261–268.

Zimmerman, M., Copeland, L., Shope, J., & Dielman, T. (1997). A longitudinal study of self-esteem: Implications for adolescent development. *Journal of Youth & Adolescence, 26*, 117–141.

Zoldbrod, A. P., & Dockett, L. (2002). *Sex talk: Uncensored exercises for exploring what really turns you on.* Oakland, CA: New Harbinger Publications, Inc.

Zumoff, B., Strain, G. W., Miller, L. K., & Rosner, W. (1995). Twenty-four hour mean plasma testosterone concentration declines with age in normal premenopausal women. *Journal of Clinical Endocrinology and Metabolism, 80*, 1429–1430.

Zurbriggen, E. L., & Yost, M. R. (2004). Power, desire, and pleasure in sexual fantasies. *The Journal of Sex Research, 41*, 288–300.

Author Index

Subject Index

Printed in the United States of America